Vulval Disease

Vulval Disease

A practical guide to diagnosis and management

Edited by

C.M. Ridley

Honorary Consultant and Senior Lecturer,
St John's Institute of Dermatology, St Thomas' Hospital, London, UK

A.J. Robinson

Consultant Physician in Genitourinary Medicine and
Honorary Senior Lecturer, Mortimer Market Centre, Camden & Islington Community Health Services
NHS Trust, London, UK

J.D. Oriel

Formerly Consultant Physician in Genitourinary Medicine,
University College Hospital, London, UK

With a contribution from

G.H. Barker

Honorary Senior Lecturer in Obstetrics and Gynaecology
St George's Hospital Medical School, London, UK

A member of the Hodder Headline Group
LONDON
Co-published in the USA by Oxford University Press Inc., New York

First published in Great Britain in 2000 by
Arnold, a member of the Hodder Headline Group,
338 Euston Road, London NW1 3BH
http://www.arnoldpublishers.com

Co-published in the USA by
Oxford University Press Inc.,
198 Madison Avenue, New York, NY10016
Oxford is a registered trademark of Oxford University Press

Whilst the advice and information in this book are believed to be true and
accurate at the date of going to press, neither the authors nor the publisher
can accept any legal responsibility or liability for any errors or omissions
that may be made. In particular (but without limiting the generality of the
preceding disclaimer) every effort has been made to check drug dosages;
however, it is still possible that errors have been missed. Furthermore,
dosage schedules are constantly being revised and new side-effects
recognized. For these reasons the reader is strongly urged to consult the
drug companies' printed instructions before administering any of the drugs
recommended in this book.

British Library Cataloguing in Publication Data
A catalogue record for this book is available from the British Library

Library of Congress Cataloguing-in-Publication Data
A catalog record for this book is available from the Library of Congress

ISBN 0 340 75890 2

1 2 3 4 5 6 7 8 9 10

Commissioning Editor: Jo Koster
Project Editor: James Rabson
Production Controller: Fiona Byrne
Cover Design: Julie Delf

Typeset in 10/13 pt Sabon by Phoenix Photosetting, Chatham, Kent
Printed and bound in Spain by Mateu Cromo, Madrid

What do you think about this book? Or any other Arnold title?
Please send your comments to feedback.arnold@hodder.co.uk

CONTENTS

PREFACE

The aim of this book is to fulfil a need encountered by the dermatologist, the gynaecologist and the physician in genitourinary medicine by serving as a useful tool in the diagnosis and management of the patients encountered in the clinic. It is designed to be a practical guide rather than a pictorial 'atlas'.

In the first chapter, the principles of history-taking and examination are followed by a guide to clinical signs and symptoms, and information on topical therapy. The chapter on infections discusses their presentation and treatment, and is accompanied by separate sections dealing with screening for infection and the general management of sexually transmitted diseases. In both the chapter on infections and that on dermatological conditions, which follows it, the material has been arranged in such a way as to reflect the types of presentation met with in clinical practice. Vulvodynia, now a very common problem, is considered in a separate chapter. A chapter on non-neoplastic swellings and neoplasms is followed by one on trauma and sexual abuse as it impinges on the clinician. The final chapter, written by a gynaecologist, provides an outline of those surgical modalities available for the treatment of vulval disease and what they entail for the patient. Throughout the text, points of special importance have been gathered together and stressed.

An appendix lists suggestions for further reading of relevance in the multidisciplinary field of vulval disease.

ACKNOWLEDGEMENTS

We thank Blackwell Scientific Publications for permission to use photographs from *The Vulva*, 2nd edition (1999), edited by C.M. Ridley and S.M. Neill.

We are grateful to the many colleagues, too many to list individually, who have so generously allowed us to see some of their patients, and to those who kindly provided some of the photographs. We are also indebted to the publishers Churchill Livingstone and Baillière Tindall, to the Editor of *British Journal of Obstetrics and Gynaecology* for permission to use previously published photographs, and to Dr Joanna Koster and James Rabson for editorial help and encouragement.

NOTE

A few older photographs in this book show ungloved fingers being used in the examination. It is now recognised that clinicians should always wear gloves when examining the anogenital area.

chapter 1

GENERAL PRINCIPLES

HISTORY AND EXAMINATION

In vulval conditions, the elicitation of the history is important. Thus, one must discover whether the patient is symptomless but has noticed some apparent abnormality, whether she is itching or whether she is complaining of pain. Topical applications should be noted, as should the patient's general health and any drugs that are being taken. Many other points may be relevant, for example a personal or family history of eczema or psoriasis, or, in the case of suspected lichen sclerosus, a personal or family history of autoimmune disease; the gynaecological and obstetric history may also turn out to be important. It is often convenient to note these and other features initially on a standard protocol. The alternative is to elicit them as necessary at the time of, or following, examination. Even if the history has to be elaborated further in the light of the findings, the initial interview is vital. Not only will it establish the main burden of the complaint, but it will also establish a relationship between the patient and the doctor and pave the way for the examination.

Examining the vulva in a methodical way, and being able to assess whether or not there are abnormalities, is the prerequisite for diagnosing and treating the many causes of vulval disease, be they related to dermatological conditions, infection or malignancy. Yet these skills are not taught to medical students, and they may elude experienced doctors, because the inspection of the vulva is not included in the routine inspection of the body. This section of the book will aim to remedy that omission.

The presence of a chaperone is obviously important, particularly but not always only for male doctors. A trained nurse is ideal; sometimes the patient will wish to be accompanied by a friend or relative in addition. There should always, however, be an opportunity for the patient to speak in private; this is especially important in the case of an adolescent who comes with her mother. The examining doctor should wear clean but not sterile gloves.

The adult patient is most conveniently examined on her back with her thighs abducted and her knees flexed. Stirrups are not advised; they are uncomfortable for the patient and limiting for looking at other areas. Colposcopy, for which stirrups are necessary, will be indicated sometimes to check cervical lesions, but is not helpful in comprehensive examination of the vulva since it produces a brightly but narrowly lit field and the magnification tends to show features such as blood vessels that are irrelevant and potentially confusing. An angled adjustable lamp at the foot of the couch, with some means of magnification for detail, such as a mirror in a bracketed frame that can be angled and which may itself incorporate a light source, is satisfactory. The routine application of 5 per cent acetic acid, as used in cervical lesions, is again not indicated. It has a non-specific whitening effect that is not of diagnostic value at the vulva. It may occasionally find a use in delineating, by its textural change, an area of intraepithelial neoplasia for the purpose of placing a biopsy.

First to be considered are the mons pubis and the labia majora (Fig. 1.1). The labia majora are covered by keratinized skin, plentifully supplied with sebaceous glands, and small aggregations of sebaceous material into papules or nodules are not uncommon. They must be parted to reveal their non-hair-bearing inner aspects, the interlabial sulci, and the thin, hairless labia minora. The labia minora are very variable in size and shape, and are often somewhat pigmented. On their upper inner aspects, it is common to see sebaceous glands appearing as yellowish dots.

There is a colour change from red to pink about midway down the inner aspect of the labia minora, forming the well-defined Hart's line, which extends forwards under the clitoris, the anterior commissure and the frenulum, and posteriorly within the posterior fourchette, which is the point of union at which the labia majora and minora diminish and fuse (Fig. 1.2). Hart's line marks the change from keratinized to non-keratinized skin. The clitoris should be examined separately. Colour changes and hypertrophy should be looked for; the clitoral hood should be easily retractible, adhesions being a patho-logical finding.

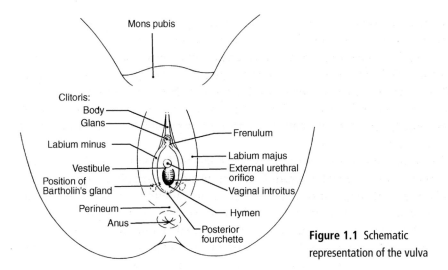

Mons pubis

Clitoris:
Body
Glans
Labium minus
Vestibule
Position of
Bartholin's gland
Perineum
Anus

Frenulum
Labium majus
External urethral
orifice
Vaginal introitus
Hymen
Posterior
fourchette

Figure 1.1 Schematic representation of the vulva

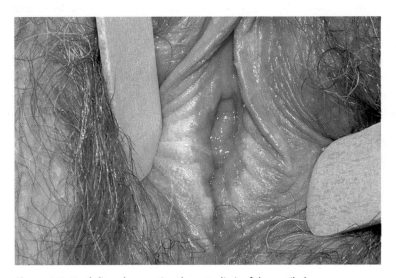

Figure 1.2 Hart's line, demarcating the outer limit of the vestibule

Inside Hart's line lies the vestibule, the inner limit of which is defined by the hymenal ring. Within the vestibule, the urethra can be seen anteriorly. The major vestibular or Bartholin's glands open into the vestibule posteriorly at the 5 o'clock and 7 o'clock positions; their openings are often marked by a degree of diffuse erythema. Small pits are sometimes to be seen dotted about; these are the openings, usually blind, of the minor vestibular glands. Frond-like, skin-coloured structures, each with a separate base, are often seen near the vaginal introitus; these are vestibular papillae (Fig. 1.3). Quite often, too, there is a diffuse velvety appearance in the vestibule that may spread out to affect in addition the whole of the inner aspects of the labia minora; this is known as vestibular papillomatosis (Fig. 1.4). It is not significantly associated with symptoms or with the human papillomavirus in spite of previous suspicions, its whitening with acetic acid is non-specific, and it may be regarded as a variant of normal. Histologically, vestibular glycogen cells appear clear after processing and may mimic the true koilocytes of HPV infection.

The perineum lies between the posterior fourchette and the anal orifice. It is smooth and hairless.

Physiological discharge and moisture vary with the menstrual cycle. Vestibular papillae and papillomatosis are mainly seen in younger women. In pregnancy, there is some engorgement and there may be varicosities. After the menopause, the tissues of the inner aspects become generally somewhat drier and thinner, although this tendency may be over-ridden to some extent by hormone replacement therapy. The hair and subcutaneous fat diminish slightly with age.

The patient is asked to turn into the left lateral position, which also affords a good view of the perineum, to enable one to inspect the anal margin, the perianal area and the skin of the natal cleft, all of which are often of relevance in vulval disease.

In many cases, it will be necessary to examine the vagina and the cervix. In some circumstances, it is necessary to carry out proctoscopy (see Ch. 2). It is of course often necessary to examine the rest of the skin, not forgetting the scalp, nails and mouth. A diagram on which to record the findings is advisable, and photographs are of value in following the progress of any given pathological condition. An account of how to describe and classify the clinical findings is given below.

EXAMINATION OF CHILDREN

It is possible to examine babies while they remain on the knee of the person with them, but it is always preferable to carry out the examination with the child on her back, in the position recommended for adults, and this is also the best way in which to look at older children. It is then usually possible, since the labia majora have not developed, to inspect all aspects of the labia minora, the clitoris and the vestibule, with little manual contact, or with none, thus minimizing disturbance to the child.

In the newborn, the clitoris and vestibule tend to be oedematous because of the influence of maternal hormones, and there may be some vaginal discharge. In

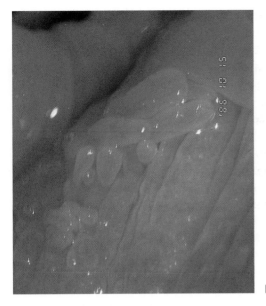

Figure 1.3 Frond-like vestibular papillae

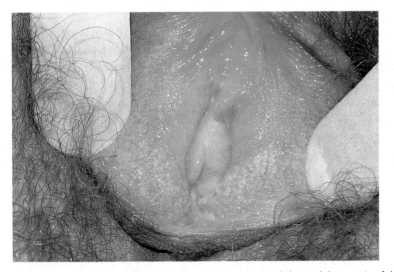

Figure 1.4 Vestibular papillomatosis. Its appearance extends beyond the margin of the vestibule to involve the inner aspect of the labia minora

infancy, a degree of cutaneous incompetence is reflected by the frequent presence of small vesicles, miliaria, related to obstruction of the sweat ducts. In childhood, the vestibule is often of a bright red colour, easily mistaken for a pathological state. The appearance of the hymen and the anal orifice must be noted with particular care when there is a question of sexual abuse. With the onset of puberty, pubic hair appears, the labia majora develop, the labia minora enlarge somewhat and the clitoris becomes larger.

INVESTIGATION

Investigations for genital infections are discussed in detail elsewhere (*see* Ch. 2). When a sexually transmitted disease is in question, the full range of screening tests must be undertaken, preferably in a genitourinary medicine clinic; the right sites must be sampled and contact tracing considered. In children, these tests are taken with special techniques and by those trained in the procedures, this applying whether or not sexual abuse is suspected. In the latter case, or wherever there are legal and forensic issues involved, further care in investigation is essential (*see* Ch. 7).

Biopsy is carried out when the diagnosis is in doubt and when management would be influenced by more exact information. Investigations relevant to the patient's general health are often indicated, for example with regard to immune status in some cases of intraepithelial neoplasia, or thyroid function in lichen sclerosus.

Following the examination, the diagnosis, and where appropriate the need for further investigation or referral, is discussed with the patient, or the parent in the case of a child. At this stage, some women like to have a friend or relative present. When appropriate, the woman should be reasssured about the absence of malignancy or infection, and questions she may have should be dealt with. Information leaflets dealing with common conditions and treatments that can be given to her to study at leisure are helpful.

The setting for the history-taking, examination and investigation will vary according to where the patient has presented herself. Referral to a multidisciplinary vulval clinic is appropriate in difficult cases.

INTRODUCTORY GUIDE TO CLINICAL SIGNS AND SYMPTOMS

SIGNS

Red lesions
This category includes angiokeratomas, Bartholin's abscess, cellulitis, eczema, erythrasma, extramammary Paget's disease, folliculitis, vulvovaginitis in a child, hidradenitis, infection superimposed on a dermatosis or trauma, lichen planus, lichen sclerosus, lichen simplex, lichenification, psoriasis, tinea, urethral caruncle,

urethral prolapse, vulval intraepithelial neoplasia and vulvitis, for example candidosis or trichomoniasis.

Pale/white lesions

Such lesions are those of lichen sclerosus, lichen simplex, lichenification, post-inflammatory depigmentation, vitiligo and vulval intraepithelial neoplasia.

Papules

Papules are found with chancre, condylomata lata, Fox–Fordyce disease, genital warts, granuloma inguinale (donovanosis), lichen planus, lichen sclerosus, lymphangiectasis, lymphogranuloma venereum, molluscum contagiosum, vestibular papillae and vulval intraepithelial neoplasia.

Pigmented lesions

Related to melanin. Melanocytic lesions are seen in lentigo, malignant melanoma and the presence of moles. Non-melanocytic lesions occur with basal cell carcinoma, genital warts, post-inflammatory pigmentation, seborrhoeic warts and vulval intraepithelial neoplasia.

Related to haemosiderin. Caruncle, lichen sclerosus, prolapse, vestibulitis are associated with haemosiderin pigmentation.

Tumours

Benign neoplasms are haemangiomas, seborrhoeic warts, skin tags, etc.

Malignant neoplasms are usually basal cell carcinoma, malignant melanoma and squamous cell carcinoma but other rarer tumours may be found.

Non-neoplastic swellings

These include, for example, cysts, varicosities and endometriomas.

Ulcers, blisters and eroded conditions

These are seen in amoebiasis, aphthous ulcers, Behçet's syndrome, bullous disorders, chancre, chancroid, fixed drug eruptions, granuloma inguinale (donovanosis), herpes simplex, herpes zoster, erosive lichen planus, eroded lichen sclerosus, mucous patches, pyoderma gangrenosum, synergistic bacterial gangrene, ulcerated tumours and vulval intraepithelial neoplasia.

Oedema

With scarring. This occurs with chronic infection, for example granuloma inguinale (donovanosis), hidradenitis or lymphogranuloma venereum.

Without scarring. This may be **acute**, as in Bartholin's abscess, candidosis, cellulitis, contact dermatitis and synergistic bacterial gangrene, or **chronic**, for example idiopathic, secondary to (repeated) cellulitis, in infection such as filariasis, in inflammatory bowel disease or after radiotherapy or surgery.

Scarring

Scarring occurs with cicatricial pemphigoid or hidradenitis, following infection such as granuloma inguinale (donovanosis) or lymphogranuloma venereum, and after radiotherapy, surgery and trauma.

Miscellaneous

Miscellaneous conditions include anatomical variants, for example ambiguous genitalia or other congenital defects, and circumcision.

SYMPTOMS

Symptoms are less reliable than signs and should never be given undue diagnostic importance as they depend upon the patient's personality, sensibility and ability to express herself. However, some conditions do tend to itch or to burn, although the two symptoms may coexist. With the caveat above, the following groupings are of some general validity.

Pruritus (itching)
- **Infections**: candidosis.
- **Dermatological conditions**, especially eczema, lichen simplex, lichenification, lichen planus, lichen sclerosus and psoriasis.
- **Neoplasia**: tumours in general, vulval intraepithelial neoplasia and extramammary Paget's disease.

Pain, soreness and burning
- **Infections**: herpes simplex, herpes zoster and trichomoniasis.
- **Dermatological conditions**: especially eczema, erosive lichen planus, lichen sclerosus and psoriasis.
- **Vulvodynia**: all variants, by definition.
- **Trauma.**

Superficial dyspareunia
This may accompany any inflammatory condition, but when given as a specific main complaint, it usually reflects vestibulitis, or lichen planus or lichen sclerosus with involvement of the perineum and/or fourchette.

TOPICAL THERAPY

This section will provide some advice on safe management when using topical treatments. The clinician should be aware of the generic names of the ingredients of proprietary preparations, should be acquainted with a few of these preparations and learn their advantages and drawbacks, and should also become accustomed to the virtues of simple non-proprietary ones. It will be helpful, moreover, to have a working knowledge of current fashions in those medications which many patients now buy themselves, whether medicinal or cosmetic, and even of what they may try by way of 'alternative' medicine. Indeed, collecting together all the preparations that the patient has used, a mélange of tubes and jars garnered from the doctor, over the counter from the pharmacist, department store or health food shop, or from friends and relations, can sometimes give a valuable insight into a patient's personality and her views on aetiology, as well as information with regard to probable adverse reactions.

It is essential to know which agents are best avoided because of their sensitizing properties, and useful to be able to advise on what remedies can be purchased without a prescription or are cheaper when bought in this way. Reference to the *British National Formulary* and the *Monthly Index of Medical Specialities* (MIMS), or to the equivalent sources outside the UK, is advised, especially for those inexperienced in dermatological therapy.

Information leaflets on common conditions should be available. These not only tell the patient something about her condition but also give her a source of reference on its treatment, and suggested régimes, for example of corticosteroid usage, can be incorporated. To a limited extent, such leaflets may be available from professional organisations, but in most cases it will be necessary, and indeed more satisfactory, to make one's own exactly to desired requirements.

SIMPLE SOOTHING APPLICATIONS

A mild solution of potassium permanganate is useful for acutely inflamed weeping and crusted areas; it is soothing and antimicrobial. It is easier to make up from the proprietary tablets (Permitabs) than from the crystals or from a concentrated solution. A strength of about 1 in 10 000, in tepid water, is a pale pink colour and is effective without leaving any unacceptable brown staining of the skin. It will, however, tend to stain a bath or washbasin, so it should be made up in a plastic bowl. The patient may sit in this for a few minutes or instead soak gauze or similar material in the fluid and apply it to the part, meanwhile protecting the surroundings with a polythene sheet. The skin is then dabbed dry with a towel. This treatment, carried out once or twice a day, should be stopped as the surface dries up. If potassium permanganate is not available, a salt-in-water solution is a useful stopgap.

BLAND EMOLLIENTS

It cannot be emphasized too strongly that in any inflammatory condition this type of preparation should always be used, often as a soap substitute and always as a moisturiser which can and indeed should be used frequently and liberally. Aqueous cream BP is safe, and cheap, and comes in tubes that can easily be carried about for daytime use. Its only drawback is that it contains a preservative that may, very rarely, irritate or cause allergic reactions. If this has happened, or if the patient has reacted badly in general to topical agents before, the parent substance, emulsifying ointment BP, is recommended; while thicker to use, it is in the main acceptable. When the patient wants to try others, there is a wide array of proprietary preparations available, the best advice being for her to sample a few. E45 cream and Diprobase are widely used. The difference in price may be marked.

Some patients like to use emollients in the bath, and those listed above can be used in this way; in the case of proprietary preparations, there are often versions made specifically for this purpose, for example E45 Wash and Balneum, designed only for the bath or shower. It is very important to warn that these applications all tend to make the bath slippery as this can be dangerous. Equally important is to make sure that the patient is not using bath salts or bubble baths, which may be irritant.

Where there is wetting from excessive discharge, sweating or incontinence of urine, and in napkin rashes, barrier preparations containing dimethicone are helpful.

ACTIVE PREPARATIONS

These are usually used as ointments rather than creams or lotions; ointments are more protective and are free of potentially allergenic preservatives.

For infections

Anti-candidal agents. Nystatin or an imidazole, for example clotrimazole or miconazole, is usually combined with a corticosteroid in the treatment of *Candida* on the skin or to prevent it. Useful preparations are Canesten-HC or Daktacort.

Antibacterial agents. The imidazoles are antibacterial. Other agents often used involve the tetracycline group (Aureocort and Trimovate) or fusidic acid (Fucibet); all these proprietary preparations contain a corticosteroid. The tetracyclines rarely sensitize but they do stain the skin and the underwear yellow, and the patient must be warned of this. An antibacterial agent alone might be used after a biopsy, the usual one being mupirocin (Bactroban). An antibacterial to be avoided is neomycin, which often sensitizes the skin.

Antiviral agents. Podophyllin for warts and aciclovir for herpes simplex are discussed elsewhere (*see* Ch. 2).

Analgesics

Prilocaine and lignocaine cream (Emla) is used before a biopsy but is not recommended as a general analgesic as it sensitizes. Lignocaine (Xylocaine) rarely sensitises; the 2 per cent gel is relatively ineffective, but the 5 per cent ointment is useful in vulvodynia.

Corticosteroids

Topical corticosteroids play an important part in topical therapy because of their anti-inflammatory and antipruritic action. When they are used judiciously, local and systemic side-effects are not a problem.

It is customary and convenient to group these substances as being mild (e.g. hydrocortisone), moderately potent (e.g. clobetasone butyrate 0.05 per cent [Eumovate]), potent (e.g. betamethasone 17-valerate 0.1 per cent [Betnovate]) and very potent (clobetasol propionate 0.05 per cent [Dermovate]). They are used alone, or sometimes in combination with an antimicrobial agent.

For napkin rashes, hydrocortisone will suffice, and stronger preparations may lead to adverse effects. In other age groups, the stronger preparations are safe to use if care is taken; unfortunately, the package inserts warn against their use in the genital area, and it must be explained to the patient that there is no danger if they are used correctly. It is useful to bear in mind that one 'finger-tip unit' is about 0.5 g and will suffice for one application.

Severe eczema and psoriasis need a moderately potent or potent corticosteroid to achieve control. When there is much lichenification, a very potent one is called for, and the amount used should be monitored; 30 g in 3 months is generally agreed to be safe, used daily and then less often in a reducing régime, and this aim is usually easily achieved as its effect is so powerful. For maintenance, the choice lies between continuing the same application but less frequently, or switching to a weaker one. A similar regime is used in lichen sclerosus.

It is wise to acquaint oneself with one or two proprietary ointments from each group.

Anti-pruritic measures

Pruritus, or itching, is a frequent accompaniment of many benign and even malignant conditions, the nature of which must be sought. When it arises as a symptom with no visible cause on apparently normal skin, this is no exception since it rapidly results in the thickening of lichen simplex. The appropriate diagnosis and treatment of these conditions will alleviate the symptoms.

Corticosteroids play an important part in treating pruritus. However, when they are proving ineffective, are not suitable for the underlying disorder or are being used to excess, the increased use of bland emollients or of such time-honoured remedies as phenol 1 per cent in calamine or zinc cream or ointment may be useful. Except in urticaria, oral antihistamines help itching only by virtue of their soporific effect. Non-sedating antihistamines are therefore of no value in this situation. Of the others, hydroxyzine, usually given at night, is particularly beneficial since it has a mild anxiolytic effect; resistance to conventional treatment is often related to a degree of anxiety.

KEY POINTS

1 Examine the patient methodically and thoroughly, remembering to include the perianal area.
2 Remember that it is often necessary also to examine the rest of the skin, the mouth, the vagina and the cervix.
3 Take note of the morphological nature of any abnormalities present; this is essential in making a diagnosis.
4 Remember the safety and efficacy of bland topical applications.
5 Become familiar with a small number of topical corticosteroids, ranging from mild to high potency.

chapter 2

VULVAL INFECTIONS

SCREENING FOR GENITAL INFECTIONS

EXAMINATION OF THE CERVIX AND VAGINA

The presence of discharge on the vulva should be noted. In many cases, it will be necessary to examine the vagina and the cervix even in the absence of discharge.

Ideally, the Cusco bivalve speculum should be warmed before insertion into the vagina. The speculum is introduced at an oblique angle and turned gently to the horizontal position. If the cervix cannot be visualized, the speculum should be removed and a finger gently inserted into the vagina to identify the position of the cervix. Once the cervix has been visualized, the speculum can be secured in order to leave both hands free to take appropriate swabs for an infection screen. Note during the examination:

● Vaginal discharge	consistency, colour and smell
● Mucosa of the vaginal walls	for erythema, ulceration and adherence of discharge
● Cervical discharge	clear, mucopurulent or purulent
● Cervix	the position of the squamo-columnar junction; and the mucosal surface

EXAMINATION OF THE ANUS AND RECTUM

Where intraepithelial neoplasia, perianal warts or unexplained perianal itching is present, investigation with proctoscopy is indicated. The proctoscope should be lubricated with saline or water and inserted with the patient in the left lateral position. Any rectal mucosal lesions or inflammation should be noted. The use of a paediatric proctoscope is appropriate if conditions such as skin tags, haemorrhoids or fissures are present and causing discomfort.

It is important to examine the rest of the skin, not forgetting the scalp, axillae, nails and mouth. A drawing of the body on which to record the findings is desirable. Photographs are of value to follow the progress in any given pathological condition.

TESTS FOR INFECTION

Ideally, the most appropriate transport medium and swabs to obtain the best results should be discussed with the microbiology department.

Skin sites

Swabs may be taken from skin sites suspected of infection. It is advisable to use specimen kits with Amies transport medium when taking samples from the genital skin.

When erythrasma is suspected, examination under Wood's light is useful in demonstrating the typical coral-red fluorescence; otherwise, scrapings taken with a blade and put into a commercially available packet lined with black paper can be sent away to the laboratory for staining and microscopy and/or culture.

In the case of tinea, scrapings may be examined in the clinic under low or high power microscopy after maceration in 10 per cent potassium hydroxide, or sent away in the same fashion for microscopy and culture.

Vagina and cervix

Plastic loops are the most appropriate for sampling vaginal discharge for microscopy. Samples should be taken by placing the loop or swab in the posterior fornix and sweeping it along the lateral vaginal wall. The sample can be spread directly on to a microscope slide for Gram staining (Fig. 2.1). A sample taken from the posterior fornix (high vaginal swab) can be placed in Amies transport medium.

Tests that can be requested are:

- microscopy to look for clue cells, trichomonads and hyphae/spores;
- culture for *Candida* species and *Trichomonas vaginalis*.

There is no value in identifying organisms such as *Gardnerella vaginalis* and mycoplasmas as these can be normal commensals.

The pH of vaginal fluid is checked by collecting a sample on a plastic loop and applying it to narrow-range pH paper (Fig. 2.2). The normal pH of the vagina is 3.5–4.5 in an adult or post-pubescent female. A sample of discharge can also be placed on a microscope slide and mixed with a drop of 10 per cent potassium hydroxide solution (KOH), which in the presence of bacterial vaginosis produces a characteristic fishy smell. This is called a 'KOH' or 'whiff' test, and together with the pH, forms one of the four criteria for the diagnosis of bacterial vaginosis.

Before taking cervical samples, the cervix should be cleaned, with a large cotton-tipped swab (colpette) or gauze held in sponge forceps, to remove vaginal and excess cervical secretions. This avoids contamination of the cervical specimens with vaginal material. A plastic loop can be placed in the cervical os to collect a sample, which is placed onto a microscope slide and spread thinly for Gram staining. The loop can then be smeared across a selective culture medium plate for the identification of *Neisseria gonorrhoeae*. If microscopy and direct

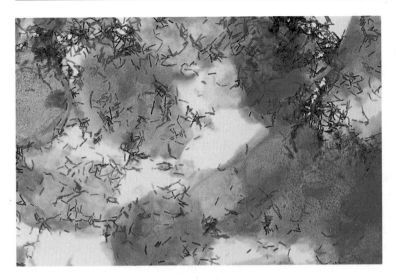

Figure 2.1 Gram stain showing normal vaginal flora

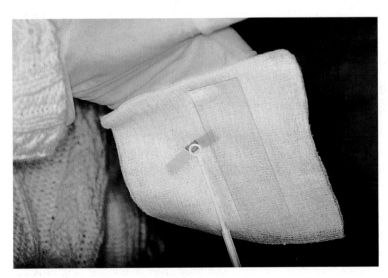

Figure 2.2 Testing the pH of vaginal discharge

culture plates are not available, a swab should be rotated in the endocervix and then placed in Amies transport medium. The specimen must be sent to the laboratory as quickly as possible to ensure the best identification rate; gonococci are fragile and die quickly.

A further sample should be taken for the detection of *Chlamydia trachomatis*. Kits are usually supplied with appropriate swabs. It is important to read the manufacturer's instructions. Most instructions accompanying kits suggest rotating the swab in the cervical canal for at least 10 seconds. If there is cervical ectopy, the swab should, in addition, be swept around the squamo-columnar junction.

If a diagnosis of genital herpes (herpes simplex virus [HSV]) is suspected, a swab can be taken from the cervical canal and placed in the appropriate viral transport medium. If there is a suspicion of human papillomavirus infection (HPV) of the cervix or vagina, washing the area with 5 per cent acetic acid should enable warts, including subclinical HPV infection, to be seen as acetowhite areas. Acetowhiteness is, however, a non-specific finding and may indicate pathology other than wart infection. If suspicious vaginal or cervical lesions are seen with or without the aid of acetic acid, colposcopic examination is recommended.

Rectum

The rectum is often a reservoir for gonorrhoea. *C. trachomatis* can also infect the rectum, giving rise to non-specific rectal symptoms.

Sampling for culture for *N. gonorrhoeae* can be carried out 'blind' in the absence of symptoms rather than by using the proctoscope. If proctoscopy is undertaken, the swab should be passed beyond the tip of the proctoscope before the sample is taken from rectal mucosa. The sample may be plated directly on to selective gonococcal medium or placed in Amies transport medium for transport to the laboratory.

Pharynx

Throat swabs may be indicated in patients with oropharyngeal symptoms or when the patient has been in contact with a person infected with gonorrhoea. A swab should be taken from the posterior fauces and placed in Stuart's transport medium.

Urethra

Urethral samples are recommended for the diagnosis of gonorrhoea. In a small number of cases, anterior vaginal wall pressure may result in discharge exuding from the urethra and a sample can be taken from this discharge; otherwise, a small plastic loop can be placed in the urethal orifice to collect a sample to be plated for the microscopy and culture of *N. gonorrhoeae*. A sample can also be taken to identify *C. trachomatis*.

Genital ulcers

In all cases of genital ulceration, an infective cause should be excluded. The clinical examination may give important information and it should be noted whether the ulcers are:

- multiple or single
- large or small
- painful
- associated with oedema
- associated with lymphadenopathy
- associated with oral ulceration.

The characteristics of the base and edge of the ulcer and whether there is surrounding erythema, evidence of scratching and superficial fissuring should also be documented. Infective causes include HSV, herpes zoster and cytomegalovirus.

To take a viral culture, pressure should be applied to the ulcer with a cotton- or dacron-tipped swab. This is likely to be painful, and patients should be warned in advance. Swabs should be transferred to the appropriate transport medium, squeezed out and discarded. The specimen should be sent to the laboratory as soon as possible, or kept at 4°C if immediate analysis is unavailable. The results of HSV culture may take up to 1 week. Other methods of diagnosis include direct immunofluorescence and antigen detection, but these are not in widespread use and have not been well evaluated.

Bartholin's gland
Bartholin's gland can be examined by inserting a finger into the vagina and moving it laterally behind and internal to the labium minus. By gently massaging the area, secretions can be expressed as far as the orifices of the duct and then collected on a swab and sent in Amies transport medium to the laboratory.

SYNDROMES OF GENITAL INFECTION

VULVAL ULCERATION/LYMPHADENOPATHY

This syndrome is predominantly the result of infection, but may have other causes, for example vulval carcinoma.

Genital herpes
In Western countries, genital herpes is the most common cause of genital ulceration, and serological studies suggest that asymptomatic infections are even more common than symptomatic cases. During the past three decades, the disease has become increasingly common.

Aetiology. HSV causes genital herpes. There are two types: HSV1 causes more than 90 per cent of orolabial herpes, and HSV2 about half of genital herpes. The two types are not therefore entirely site specific; about 50 per cent of first attacks of genital herpes are caused by HSV1, mostly contracted through oral sex. Either virus can be introduced into genital epithelial cells through sexual contact. Soon afterwards, it spreads along sensory nerves to the dorsal root ganglia, where it becomes latent. Latency persists indefinitely, and reactivation, leading to further attacks of disease, can occur at any time; these may be provoked by factors such as intercourse, menstruation and psychological stress, but are often inexplicable.

Clinical features. Infection in women follows vaginal or orogenital contact with an individual shedding the virus. The source contact may have obvious lesions, but in many cases the partner has minimal or no signs of infection. The incubation period for a first attack of genital herpes is about a week (range 2–12 days). Irritation at the site may precede the appearance of a group of vesicles (Fig. 2.3). These evolve into pustules, which erode to form superficial painful ulcers (Fig. 2.4), crusting and healing in 2–3 weeks. Lesions occur around the introitus, the urethra and the labia, or may involve the perineum, perianal area and thighs. Tender inguinal adenopathy occurs in about 80 per cent of patients. New lesions may appear in crops until about the 10th day, which delays healing. Cervicitis develops in up to 90 per cent of women with primary attacks of herpes, the cervix appearing red, friable or ulcerated.

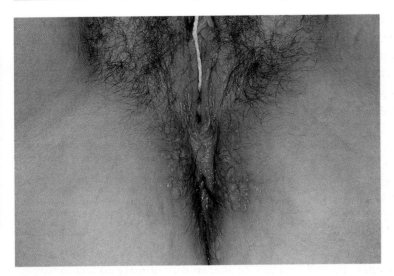

Figure 2.3 Herpes vesicles

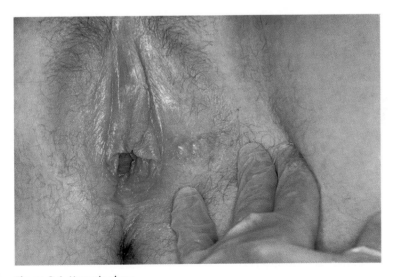

Figure 2.4 Herpetic ulcers

Patients often have systemic symptoms, which include fever, malaise and myalgia. Severe and prolonged headache may indicate the onset of aseptic meningitis, which affects one third of women with primary genital herpes. Sacral radiculitis, causing retention of urine, may also occur. The presentation of primary genital herpes varies between individuals according to their host responses. Antecedent chronic eczema makes the skin liable to a severe infection – eczema herpeticum (Fig. 2.5). In patients with altered immunity, such as pregnancy or HIV infection, herpes may run a severe and prolonged course.

About 80 per cent of women with primary infections with HSV2 develop recurrences within the year following the infection. The frequency of recurrence varies between one and six or more times a year. Some of these may simply be episodes of symptomless viral shedding, but others are symptomatic, of variable severity and lasting 10 days or more. HSV1 causes fewer symptomatic recurrences than HSV2. Cervical infection is uncommon in recurrent attacks.

Diagnosis. Painful grouped vesicles on the vulva are virtually diagnostic of herpes, although there are other causes of painful erosions (Table 2.1); virus culture is the most sensitive laboratory test. Specimens of vesicle fluid, or ones taken from the base of an ulcer, are placed into transport medium. In a first attack, it is advisable to sample the cervix as well. In the laboratory, the specimens are inoculated into a suitable cell line, incubated and examined regularly. If the inoculum is large, a cytopathic effect will be apparent in 1–7 days. The viral isolates can be confirmed, and typed if desired, by immunofluorescence.

Table 2.1 Differential diagnosis of genital herpes

Chancroid
Primary syphilis
Traumatic ulcers
Contact dermatitis
Other bullous/erosive dermatoses

Treatment. Women with genital herpes will need counselling to enable them to learn to live with the condition. Aciclovir is the best drug for specific treatment. For a first attack, 200 mg five times a day orally has a marked effect in reducing the duration and severity of symptoms.

Patients with mild recurrences need only symptomatic treatment, but if attacks are severe, a course of aciclovir can be given for each episode, beginning treatment as early as possible. Women with frequent recurrences benefit from suppressive aciclovir therapy. Many avoid attacks by taking 200 mg four times a day, and it may be possible to reduce this to 200 mg twice daily. Such courses should continue for 6–12 months at a time.

Famciclovir is similar to aciclovir but needs to be taken less often. For a first episode of genital herpes, the dose is 250 mg three times a day for 5 days. Similarly valciclovir may be used instead of aciclovir.

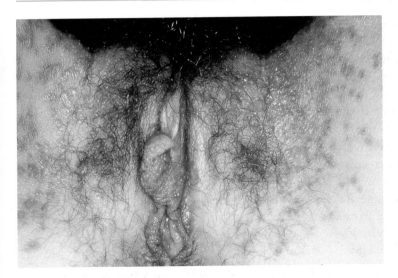

Figure 2.5 Eczema herpeticum

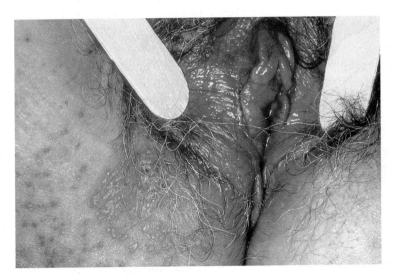

Figure 2.6 Herpes zoster

Herpes zoster

This is caused by the varicella-zoster virus. Vulval lesions appear if the S3 dermatome is affected. The rash is preceded by local pain or paraesthesiae. It is unilateral, with vesicles against a background of erythema (Fig. 2.6). After a few days, crusts form and separate without scarring. The eruption is painful at the time, and a few patients experience post-herpetic neuralgia after the attack.

Herpes zoster may occur at any stage of an HIV infection, when it is likely to be more severe and prolonged.

Diagnosis and treatment. The diagnosis of a unilateral painful vesicular rash is usually easy; if necessary, it can be confirmed by virus culture. If the disease is severe, for example in elderly or immunocompromised patients, aciclovir 800 mg five times a day by mouth is helpful if given early in an attack and should be continued until there have been no new lesions for 48 hours.

Chancroid

Aetiology. Chancroid is an acute sexually transmitted infection caused by *Haemophilus ducreyi*. It has become uncommon in the Western world, although local outbreaks may occur, but in tropical and subtropical countries, particularly parts of Africa, Asia and Latin America, it is the most common cause of genital ulceration.

Clinical features. The incubation period is 3–10 days. Small, tender papules appear, which soon break down to form ragged, tender, non-indurated ulcers (Fig. 2.7). These may be single (a) or multiple (b); the majority occur on the labia, perineum and perianal areas. Inguinal adenitis develops in up to 50 per cent of women with chancroid, and a mass of these glands may suppurate and form abscesses. These may rupture spontaneously, leaving fistulae. Secondary infection with fusospiro-chaetal organisms may sometimes lead to a rapidly destructive phagedena ('eating of flesh'); a concomitant infection with HIV may have a similar effect.

Diagnosis. The differential diagnosis is from other causes of genital ulceration/lymphadenopathy syndrome, particularly syphilis and genital herpes. Their clinical differentiation may be difficult, and one of these usually coexists in 10 per cent of cases of chancroid. A dark-field examination for *Treponema pallidum* and serological tests for syphilis are essential. A Gram-stained smear may show groups of Gram-negative streptobacillary organisms, but this is an insensitive procedure, and the isolation of *H. ducreyi* from the ulcers or pus on special media is preferable, although even this may be difficult owing to the fastidious nature of the organisms.

Treatment. *H. ducreyi* has become resistant to many antimicrobial agents. At present, the drug of choice is erythromycin base or stearate, 500 mg four times a day orally for 7 days.

Syphilis

Aetiology. Syphilis is a chronic systemic sexually transmitted disease caused by *T. pallidum*. This is a slender spiral organism best seen by dark-field microscopy

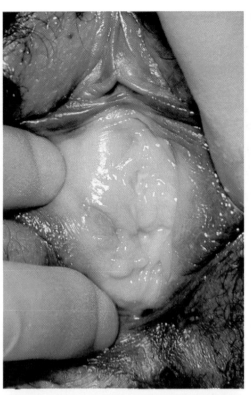

(a)

Figure 2.7 Chancroid

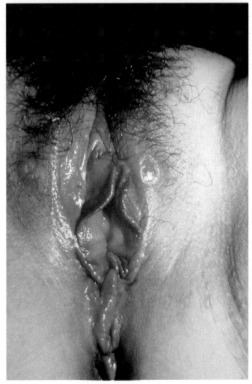

(b)

of a fresh wet preparation, in which it can be seen to undergo rotary movements and angulation. The organism has not been propagated *in vitro*.

The incidence of syphilis in adults declined markedly after the Second World War and has remained low in western Europe since then. In the USA, Russia and eastern European countries, there has been an increase over the past decade, related to promiscuity and drug addiction among poor people in conurbations. In underdeveloped countries, notably Africa, syphilis is common.

Clinical features. After an incubation period of 9–90 days, the initial lesion appears, usually on the genitals, as a small papule, which enlarges and ulcerates to form a primary chancre. A classical (Hunterian) chancre is indurated (Fig. 2.8) and painless unless secondarily infected. In women, chancres appear on the labia, on the fourchette and sometimes at the anus or cervix. They are often multiple, and without treatment heal in up to 6 weeks. In the majority of cases, the regional lymph nodes enlarge within a week of the appearance of the chancre; they are usually painless, firm and smooth.

Secondary syphilis appears 3–6 weeks after the primary chancre. This is a systemic disease. The main signs are malaise, fever, rashes or lesions of the skin and mucous membranes, as well as widespread lymphadenopathy. The rashes – macular, papular, papulo-squamous or pustular – may affect any area, including the vulva. Condylomata lata (Fig. 2.9) are classically perivulval and perianal; they are soft and spongy, with flat tops that may become eroded. Mucous patches usually appear at the same time. These are painless eroded areas affecting the labia minora and mouth.

With exacerbations and remissions, secondary syphilis may last for up to 2 years, but all signs of disease eventually disappear, although the patient remains infectious, with positive serological tests; this state is known as latent syphilis. The various manifestations of late syphilis develop in one third of patients after 5–20 years, but these are now very rare.

Diagnosis. Syphilis is notorious for resembling other diseases. Chancres of the vulva must be differentiated from other forms of ulceration, including genital herpes, pyogenic lesions and, in developing countries, chancroid, lympho-granuloma venereum and donovanosis. Clinical diagnosis of the aetiology of vulval ulcers is unreliable, and laboratory investigation is essential; it must be remembered that more than one cause may be present. The vulval lesions of secondary syphilis may resemble many dermatoses. Mucous patches may be confused with genital herpes, and condylomata lata with genital warts.The laboratory diagnosis of early syphilis depends on the dark-field examination of fluid expressed from lesions, or obtained by gland puncture, for characteristic motile treponemes. Alternatively, the organisms may be stained with a fluorescent-labelled conjugate specific for *T. pallidum*. Serological tests for syphilis are essential. Those commonly used are (Table 2.2):

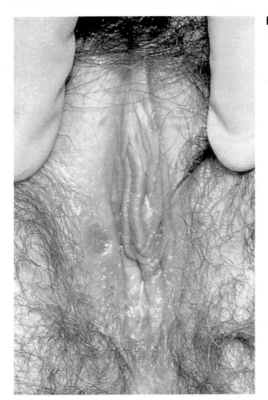

Figure 2.8 Primary chancre

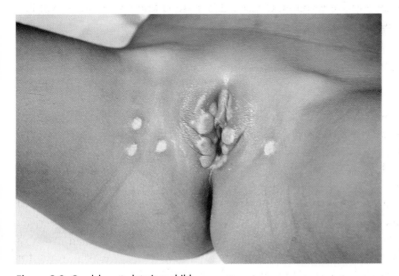

Figure 2.9 Condylomata lata in a child

1 **Non-specific tests:** the Venereal Disease Research Laboratory (VDRL) and Rapid Plasma Reagin (RPR) tests;
2 **Specific tests:** the Fluorescent Treponemal Absorbed (FTA-ABS) test and the Treponema Pallidum Haemagglutination Assay (TPHA).

Table 2.2 Percentage sensitivity of serological tests in untreated syphilis

	Primary	Secondary	Latent
VDRL/RPR	60–90	99–100	70–90
FTA-ABS	85–100	100	95–100
TPHA	65–85	99–100	95–100

For abbreviations, see text.

Treatment. Penicillin remains the antimicrobial agent of choice. For primary, secondary and early latent syphilis, the following are recommended:

- procaine penicillin 1200 units daily intramuscularly for 10 days; or
- benzathine penicillin G 2.4 million units as a single intramuscular injection.

Patients who are allergic to penicillin may be given:

- tetracycline hydrochloride 500 mg four times a day orally for 15 days, or doxycycline 100 mg twice daily for 15 days; or if pregnant,
- erythromycin 500 mg four times a day orally for 15 days.

Experience of treating syphilis with non-penicillin regimes is limited, and the post-treatment review of such patients must be careful. Patients often experience fever and malaise a few hours after their first dose of antimicrobial medication; a primary chancre may enlarge, or secondary signs appear for the first time. No special treatment is necessary, and such reactions do not recur.

Lymphogranuloma venereum

Aetiology. This sexually transmitted disease is caused by specific serovars (L1–3) of *Chlamydia trachomatis* that predominantly affect lymphoid tissue. It is endemic in sub-Saharan Africa and South America but is rare in Western countries.

Clinical features. The incubation period is usually 3–5 days but may be longer. The primary lesion is a small, painless papule or ulcer that heals rapidly and may escape notice. In women, it occurs most commonly on the fourchette, labia and cervix. Lymphadenopathy develops several weeks later (Fig. 2.10). If the primary lesion was on the labia, the inguinal glands become enlarged and painful, and may suppurate and form sinuses. Healing is slow, even with treatment, and there is much scarring. If the infection involves the rectal lymphatics, an 'anorectal syndrome' develops. This begins as an acute proctocolitis, and perirectal abscesses and fistulae may follow (Fig. 2.11). Vulval elephantiasis with ulceration (esthiomène) is caused by chronic active infection, with lymphatic obstruction.

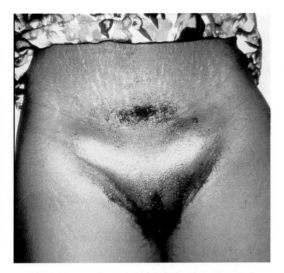

Figure 2.10 Lymphogranuloma venereum: adenopathy

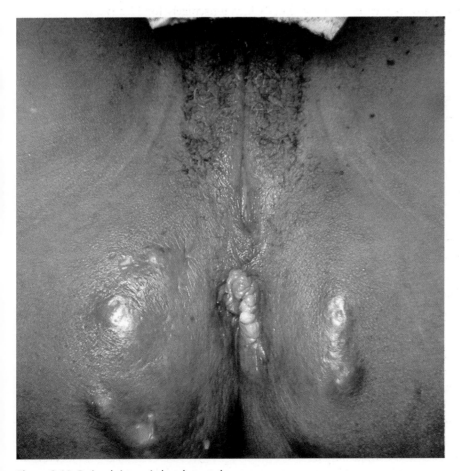

Figure 2.11 Perianal sinuses in lymphogranuloma venereum

Diagnosis. Lymphogranuloma venereum (LGV) must be differentiated from other causes of genital ulceration/lymphadenopathy. Syphilis serology must be performed. The best specific test is cell culture of aspirated pus for *C. trachomatis*. The LGV complement fixation test is widely used, a titre of over 64 being confirmatory if characteristic signs are present.

Treatment. LGV responds well to tetracyclines; for example, tetracycline hydrochloride 2 g per day in divided doses for 2–3 weeks is a common regime, which may need to be prolonged. An equivalent dose of erythromycin is a possible alternative. Abscesses should be aspirated to avoid sinus formation.

Donovanosis

Donovanosis, formerly called granuloma inguinale, is a sexually transmitted disease caused by *Calymmatobacterium granulomatis*, a Gram-negative encapsulated rod of uncertain genus. It occurs mostly in subtropical countries such as India, Brazil, the West Indies and parts of South Africa.

Clinical features. The incubation period is 2–4 weeks. The first lesions are papular, occuring on the labia and perivulval area. These break down to form deep irregular ulcers with a granular base, which may become extensive and very destructive (Fig. 2.12). Regional lymphadenopathy does not occur. The ulcers are unlikely to heal without treatment.

Diagnosis. The differential diagnosis is from other kinds of genital ulceration, particularly syphilis and chancroid. Other infections, including HIV, are not uncommon in donovanosis. The laboratory diagnosis depends on identifying *Calymmatobacterium granulomatis* in tissue smears stained with Giemsa, which show intracellular 'Donovan bodies' (Fig. 2.13). The organisms have not been cultured on conventional media. Histology is valuable in order to exclude malignancy.

Treatment. Donovanosis responds well to tetracycline hydrochloride 500 mg four times daily, or an equivalent dose of erythromycin, given orally for 2–3 weeks.

Figure 2.12 Donovanosis

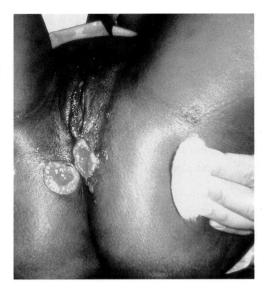

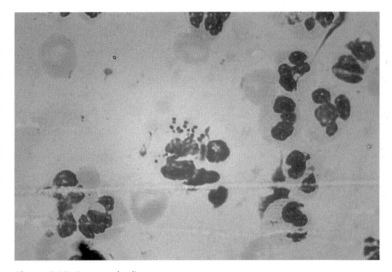

Figure 2.13 Donovan bodies

Amoebiasis

Aetiology. *Entamoeba histolytica* exists in two forms – the motile trophozoite and the cyst – the former being the pathogenic form, living in the lumen and/or walls of the colon. Infection is worldwide, commonly occurring in tropical and subtropical countries. Ulceration of the female genitalia is an unusual complication.

Clinical features. Lesions begin as cutaneous abscesses of the vulva or perineum that rupture to form painful irregular ulcers with a sloughing base (Fig. 2.14). There may be regional lymphadenopathy, and intestinal amoebiasis is usually present.

Diagnosis. Vulval amoebiasis must be distinguished from other members of the genital ulcer/lymphadenopathy syndrome. The specific diagnosis may be made by identifying motile amoebae in the purulent exudate from the ulcers or cervix; trophozoites or cysts may be found in fresh stool specimens.

Treatment. Metronidazole 800 mg three times a day for 5 days is an effective treatment. A course of diloxanide furonate, 500 mg three times daily for 10 days, should follow in order to clear the cysts from the bowel.

VULVOVAGINAL INFECTIONS

Candidosis

Aetiology. Vulvovaginal yeast infections are common. *Candida albicans* causes 90 per cent and other *Candida* species the remainder. Microscopy shows the organisms as ovoid budding yeasts and pseudohyphae. Endogenous yeasts are ubiquitous; asymptomatic vaginal colonization occurs in 15 per cent of women. The causes of symptomatic disease include pregnancy, diabetes, high-oestrogen oral contraceptives, systemic antimicrobial therapy and immunosuppression; vulvovaginal candidosis may occasionally be an early indication of HIV disease. In some cases of recurrent infection, no predisposing cause can be identified.

Clinical features. The vulva and vagina are involved together. The cardinal symptom is pruritus, and burning, dysuria and vaginal discharge may also be present. The vulva shows erythema, scaling, excoriation and swelling. The vagina is inflamed, and a curdy discharge is often present (Fig. 2.15a). The pH is under

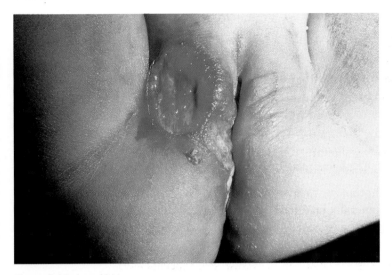

Figure 2.14 Amoebiasis

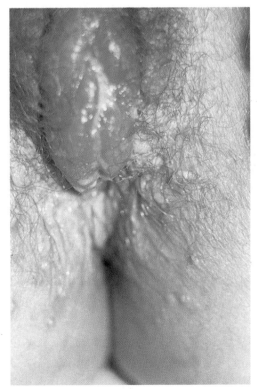

Figure 2.15 (a) Candidal vulvitis with oedema, erythema and profuse discharge.

4.5, and amine tests are negative. Candidosis may complicate other infections, such as herpes; equally, candidosis with fissuring may be confused with herpes (Fig. 2.15b).

Diagnosis. The diagnosis of candidosis may be made by microscopy of a specimen of discharge mixed with saline or 10 per cent potassium hydroxide, to show yeast cells or pseudohyphae; alternatively, a Gram-stained smear shows these as intensely Gram-positive (Fig. 2.16). Neither of these methods has more than 50 per cent of the sensitivity of culture, performed on Sabouraud's or a similar medium. The urine should always be tested to exclude glycosuria.

Treatment. Symptomatic vulvovaginal candidosis requires treatment. The imidazoles are generally preferred, for example clotrimazole pessaries 100 mg at night for 6 nights, or 500 mg as a single pessary. The other imidazoles are equally effective, and cure rates of 90 per cent may be expected. Acute candidosis may also be treated with a single dose of fluconazole 150 mg orally.

Recurrent infections are a difficult problem for some women. Once obvious provoking factors have been excluded, the best approach is probably intermittent prophylactic therapy. A single 500 mg clotrimazole pessary can be used empirically at the onset of symptoms. Alternatively, a 500 mg pessary may be used, perhaps before or after menstruation, for several weeks. Intermittent oral fluconazole may be used in the same way. Such therapy is suppressive rather than curative.

Bacterial vaginosis

Aetiology. Bacterial vaginosis (formerly called non-specific vaginitis) is included here as the most common cause of abnormal vaginal discharge. It results from a disturbance of the vaginal flora involving a loss of the normal lactobacilli and overgrowth with Gardnerella and anaerobes. Its cause is unknown; although it is associated with sexual activity, it is not regarded as a sexually transmitted disease.

Clinical features. Women complain of a vaginal discharge that smells unpleasant, and sometimes of mild vulvovaginal irritation. The vulva and vaginal epithelia appear normal, but there is a milky vaginal discharge. The vaginal pH is over 4.5, and a fishy, amine odour can be smelt when the secretions are mixed with 10 per cent potassium hydroxide.

Diagnosis. A wet mount or Gram-stained smear reveals 'clue cells', which are vaginal epithelial cells whose edges are obscured by bacteria. No lactobacilli, but many other bacteria, are seen. Culture is not necessary for diagnosis.

Treatment. Metronidazole 400 mg twice a day for 5 days is usually curative. A course of 2 per cent clindamycin cream applied intravaginally for 7 days is also effective. Recurrences after treatment are common.

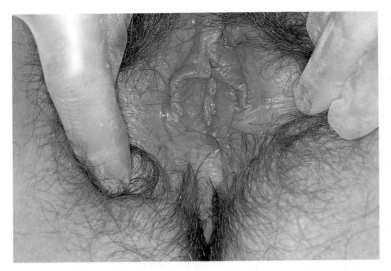

Figure 2.15 (b) Candidal vulvitis with fissuring.

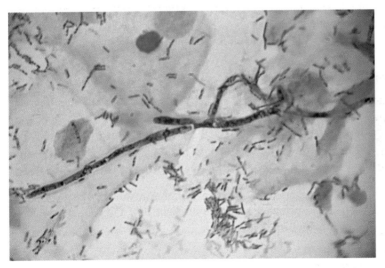

Figure 2.16 *Candida albicans*: yeast cells and hyphae

Trichomoniasis

Aetiology. This is a sexually transmitted disease caused by *Trichomonas vaginalis*, a motile, flagellated protozoon (Fig. 2.17). It infects the genital tract exclusively, and may persist for months or even years if untreated. Concomitant infection with other organisms, notably *N. gonorrhoeae*, is common.

Clinical features. Up to 50 per cent of women infected by *Trichomonas vaginalis* are symptomless, the remainder complaining of vaginal discharge, dysuria and vulval irritation. Examination classically shows acute vulvovaginitis with a purulent, frothy and malodorous discharge (Fig. 2.18); in severe infections, there may be punctate haemorrhages on the cervix ('strawberry cervix').

Diagnosis. The simplest technique is microscopy of a drop of vaginal fluid mixed with saline. The irregular jerky movements of the organisms can be seen at low power, and at higher power the flagellae can be identified. The sensitivity of microscopy is 50–75 per cent; culture in nutrient liquid media gives better results. Trichomonads can also be identified in smears stained by Giemsa or Papanicolaou, and a fluorescent-labelled antibody stain is also available.

Treatment. Metronidazole is the drug of choice. Single oral doses of 2 g, or a course of 200 mg three times a day for 7 days, are equally effective. Sexual partners should be similarly treated. Metronidazole should be avoided if possible during the first 3 months of pregnancy, but after this it is safe.

INFECTIVE PERIGENITAL RASHES

Oxyuriasis

Aetiology. Infection by *Enterobius vermicularis* (threadworms) is common, particularly in children. The worms inhabit the large bowel and lay eggs on the perianal skin during the night; these may then be ingested by another person, or the larvae may re-enter the subject's own anal canal.

Clinical features. Pruritus ani is a common symptom, but vulval irritation and vulvovaginitis may also occur, and worms may be found in the vagina.

Diagnosis and treatment. Threadworms may be seen around the anus or between the labia. The ova may be identified by microscopy after the application of adhesive tape.

General measures to prevent self-infection are important, the hands and nails being thoroughly scrubbed before meals and after urination and defecation. If possible, a bath or a shower in the morning is advisable. Anthelmintics are effective, and all family members should be treated. Piperazine salts may be given daily for 7 days, single dose preparations also being available.

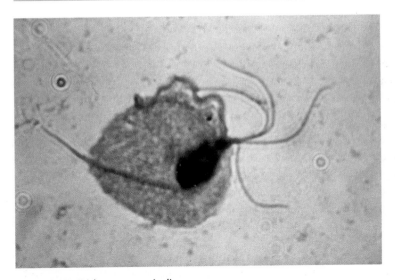

Figure 2.17 *Trichomonas vaginalis*

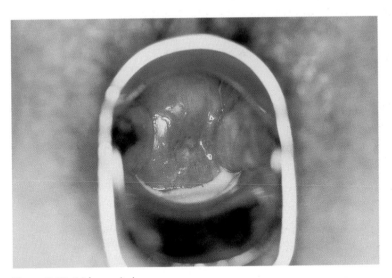

Figure 2.18 Trichomoniasis

Pediculosis pubis

Aetiology. This sexually transmitted disease is caused by the crab louse *Phthirus pubis*. This wingless insect, flattened dorsoventrally and 1–2 mm long, has two of its six legs modified for grasping hair (Fig. 2.19), and adult lice feed by sucking blood from their hosts. The eggs (nits) are cemented to the hairs near their roots.

Clinical features. The incubation period is about 4 weeks. Infestation may be symptomless, but patients usually present with vulval irritation or because they have seen the insects moving. The pubic, vulval and perianal areas are most often affected, and both adult lice and nits will be present (Fig. 2.20). Non-genital hairy areas such as the axillae, eyebrows and eyelashes may be affected, but not the scalp.

Treatment. Tests for other sexually transmitted diseases should be performed before treatment is commenced. Malathion is effective; an aqueous 0.5 per cent lotion should be applied to pubic and perianal areas for 12 hours or overnight. Other sites should be inspected and, if necessary, treated. A second treatment is advisable after 7 days to kill lice emerging from the surviving eggs. Alcoholic lotions are not recommended. Sexual contacts should be examined, and treated if necessary.

Figure 2.19 *Phthirus pubis*

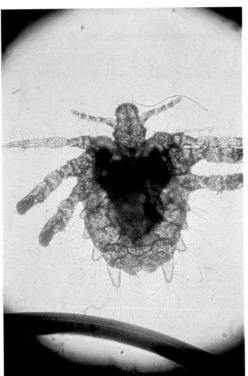

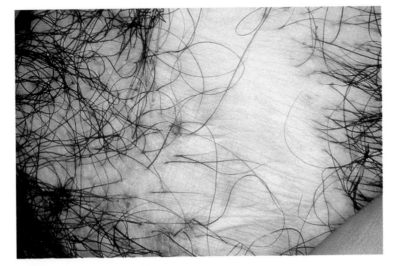

Figure 2.20 Pediculosis pubis

Tinea cruris

Aetiology. Tinea cruris is a fungal infection, usually caused by *Trichophyton rubrum* or *Epidermophyton floccosum*. Heat, humidity and tight underwear are all provoking factors.

Clinical features. Tinea presents as an irritating erythematous plaque with a raised edge, which spreads periperally and tends to clear in the centre (Fig. 2.21a and b). The groins are mostly affected, but the rash may spread to the vulva, perineum and perianal areas. There is often a focus elsewhere, usually on the feet.

Diagnosis. Microscopy of scrapings from the edge of the eruption suspended in 10 per cent potassium hydroxide may reveal fungal filaments, and the same material can be cultured. The main differential diagnoses are flexural psoriasis, erythrasma and cutaneous candidosis.

Treatment. Local applications of an imidazole cream such as clotrimazole 1 per cent may be made and continued for a week or two after clinical clearance. In hair-bearing areas, topical treatment may be unsuccessful, so oral treatment with terbinafine 250 mg daily, for 2–4 weeks is recommended.

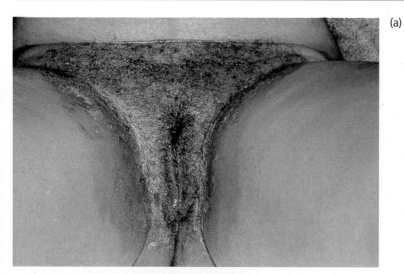
(a)

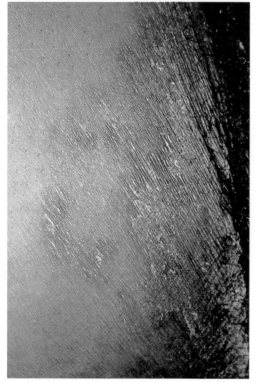
(b)

Figure 2.21 Tinea cruris: (a) Typical scaly rash. (b) Scaly edge and tendency to central clearing.

Erythrasma

Aetiology. This condition is caused by *Corynebacterium minutissimum*, which forms part of the normal skin flora but may overgrow and cause a rash in warm climates or in debilitated people.

Clinical features. Genital erythrasma affects the groins and natal cleft, where it forms an itchy eruption of brownish scaly patches (Fig. 2.22).

Diagnosis. Erythrasma must be distinguished from tinea cruris, flexural eczema and seborrhoeic dermatitis. Under Wood's light, it may show a coral-red fluorescence, and *Corynebacterium minutissimum* can be cultured on special media.

Treatment. The preferred treatment is oral erythromycin 250 mg four times a day for 2 weeks. Recurrence is common, and clotrimazole cream may be useful for long-term therapy.

PYOGENIC INFECTIONS

Gonorrhoea

Aetiology. Gonorrhoea is a common worldwide sexually transmitted disease caused by *N. gonorrhoeae*, a Gram-negative diplococcus. It is highly infectious. The risk of a woman becoming infected from a single sexual contact is unknown, but 90 per cent of the female partners of men with gonorrhoea become infected.

Clinical features. The cervix is infected in 90 per cent of cases of gonorrhoea, the urethra in 75 per cent and the rectum in 50 per cent. About 50 per cent of women with uncomplicated gonorrhoea are symptomless. The remainder complain of vaginal discharge, dysuria and vulval discomfort, but these symptoms are non-specific and may be caused by associated infections. The incubation period is up to 10 days. There are no characteristic physical signs; in some women, there is evidence of cervicitis, and pus can sometimes be expressed from the urethra (Fig. 2.23).

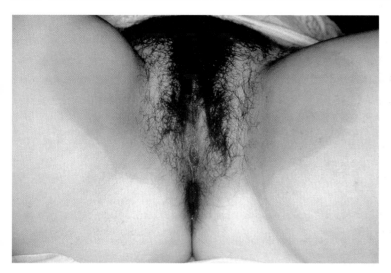

Figure 2.22 Erythrasma

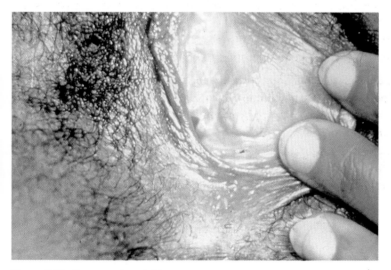

Figure 2.23 Gonococcal urethritis

The complications of gonorrhoea include periurethral abscess (Fig. 2.24) and abscesses of Bartholin's gland, but the most serious is acute salpingitis, which develops in 10–15 per cent of women. Disseminated infections may also occur.

Diagnosis. This depends entirely on the results of laboratory tests. Specimens are taken from the cervix, urethra, rectum and pharynx, high vaginal swabs being useless. Microscopy of Gram-stained specimens for Gram-negative intracellular diplococci will identify only 50 per cent of confirmed gonococcal infections of the urethra, cervix and anorectum, and is ineffective for pharyngeal specimens. Culture on selective media is much more reliable, positive results being confirmed by sugar fermentation or immunofluorescence.

Treatment. The treatment of gonorrhoea is outlined in Table 2.3.

Table 2.3 Treatment of uncomplicated gonorrhoea[a]

Level of gonococcal resistance to penicillin	Recommended therapy (single dose)
High	Ciprofloxacin 500 mg orally
	Ceftriaxone 200 mg intramuscularly
	Spectinomycin 2.0 g intramuscularly
Low	Ampicillin 2.0 g + 1.0 g oral probenecid

[a]Co-infection with *C. trachomatis* occurs in 30–50% of women with gonorrhoea, so each of the above regimes should be followed by an adequate course of a tetracycline, e.g. doxycycline 100 mg twice a day for 7 days.

Chlamydia trachomatis infection

Aetiology. *Chlamydia trachomatis* is a Gram-negative intracellular bacterium with a complex life cycle. Of its serovars, A–C cause trachoma, D–K a group of oculogenital infections that includes non-gonococcal urethritis in men and related disorders in women, and L1-3 lymphogranuloma venereum.

Clinical features. In women, the major target of infection is the columnar epithelium of the endocervix. Urethral infection is not uncommon, usually accompanying infection of the cervix, and is usually symptomless. The impact of *C. trachomatis* on the vulva is slight. Chlamydiae alone do not affect Bartholin's glands.

Diagnosis. Vulval specimens may be required from the urethra. Cell culture was the standard diagnostic test, but many laboratories now employ antigen detection or DNA amplification tests.

Treatment. The tetracyclines are widely used, for example doxycycline 100 mg twice daily for 7 days. The azalide macrolide azithromycin in a single oral dose of 1.0 g has recently been found to be highly effective.

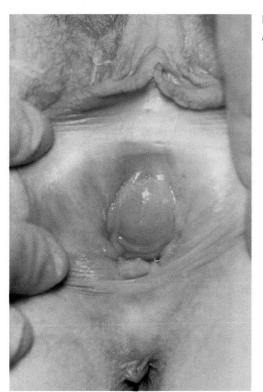

Figure 2.24 Periurethral gonococcal abscess

Septic dermatoses

Staphylococcus aureus may cause furuncles and folliculitis on the vulva (Fig. 2.25). Single furuncles are not uncommon and may recur despite treatment. Multiple furuncles may be associated with diabetes mellitus and immune deficiency. Folliculitis may follow minor trauma such as shaving the perigenital hair, and may complicate almost any variety of vulvitis or vulval dermatosis. *S. aureus* is a common cause of abscess of Bartholin's gland, others being *N. gonorrhoeae* and *Streptococcus faecalis*.

A tender swelling appears at the affected labium majus, with oedema and erythema (Fig. 2.26). The abscess may discharge spontaneously or require surgical treatment. *Streptococcus pyogenes* causes cellulitis (erysipelas) of the vulva, a spreading inflammation of the dermis that may follow fissures or operation wounds, or complicate all kinds of lymphatic obstruction.

Treatment. Minor degrees of folliculitis and single furuncles do not merit systemic treatment, but extensive folliculitis and severe furunculosis require antimicrobials. Since many staphylococci are coagulase producing, flucloxacillin 250 mg four times a day is taken for 5–7 days. A similar regimen may be used for the initial treatment of infection of Bartholin's gland pending microbiology. Oral or parenteral penicillin is rapidly effective for cellulitis; erythromycin can be substituted for those allergic to penicillin.

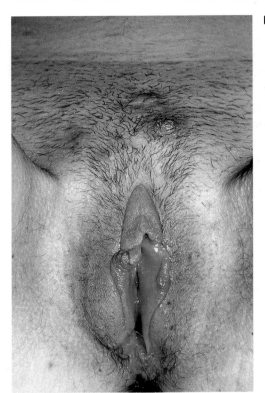

Figure 2.25 Vulval folliculitis

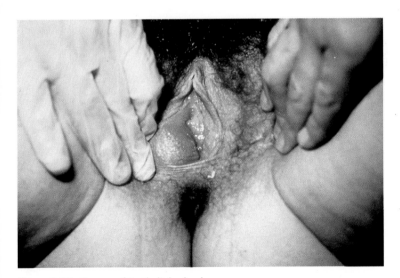

Figure 2.26 Abscess of Bartholin's gland

CONDYLOMAS AND PAPULES

Papillomavirus infections

Infection of the genital tract with HPV is a common sexually transmitted disease, comprising various types of genital wart and a large subclinical component.

Aetiology. HPV is a spherical DNA virus, 50 nm in diameter, which replicates in the nuclei of epithelial cells. It has not been propagated *in vitro*, but molecular virology has shown that there are more than 70 genotypes of the virus (Table 2.4). Those affecting the vulva may also infect the cervix.

The incidence of genital warts has markedly increased in recent years. They are most often seen in women aged 20–24 years. Genital warts are sexually transmissible, and 60 per cent of the current male partners of affected women have penile warts.

Clinical features. Vulval HPV infection may be clinical or subclinical. The clinical lesions are condylomata acuminata and papular (sessile) warts. Condylomata acuminata (Fig. 2.27) affect the fourchette and adjacent labia, the perineum, the anus, the vagina and the cervix. They are multicentric, so several areas may be affected at the same time. The condylomas are soft, fleshy and vascular, and may coalesce into large masses. They may be pigmented; vulval intraepithelial neoplasia occurs most often in these and also in some hyperkeratotic plaques. Papular warts occur on dry areas such as the labia majora; they are usually raised and multiple (Fig. 2.28). Genital warts enlarge if there is impaired immunity, as in women who are pregnant, suffering from HIV

Table 2.4 Manifestations of human papillomavirus genotypes

Genotype	Lesions
HPV 6, 11	Genital warts
HPV 16, 18, 31	Vulval intraepithelial neoplasia (VIN)
	Squamous cell carcinoma

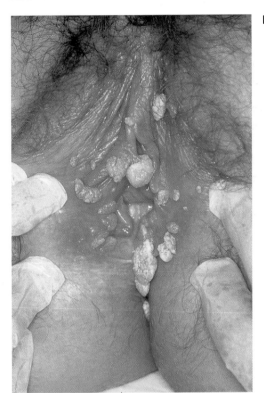

Figure 2.27 Condylomata acuminata

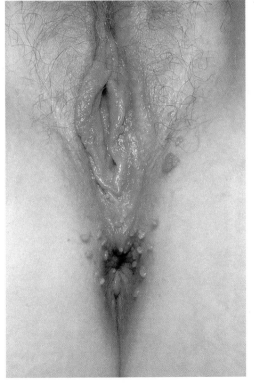

Figure 2.28 Papular warts

infection or lymphoma (Fig. 2.29), or immunosuppressed after a renal transplant. Giant condyloma is a rare tumour, locally destructive, but on the whole histologically benign. Subclinical HPV infection presents on the vulva as 'flat condylomas' – condylomata plana (Fig. 2.30).

Areas of white epithelial discontinuity can be identified after the application of 5 per cent aqueous acetic acid, particularly with the aid of a colposcope. These acetowhite areas may or may not be associated with clinically apparent warts. Any part of the vulva may be affected. It should be noted that acetowhitening is not necessarily caused by HPV infection; some dermatoses, and vestibular papillomatosis, may show a similar non-specific appearance.

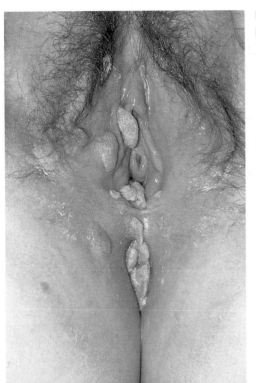

Figure 2.29 Large warts in a patient with lymphoma

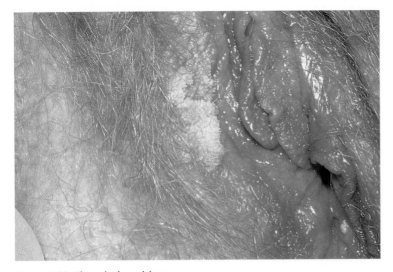

Figure 2.30 Flat vulval condylomas

Diagnosis. Vulval warts must be distinguished from fibroepithelial polyps, condylomata lata, molluscum contagiosum, other benign vulval tumours, VIN and squamous cell carcinoma. Biopsy of any atypical lesion is obviously essential. The histopathology of genital warts shows papillomatosis and acanthosis (Fig. 2.31). True koilocytes, which are large vacuolated cells present in the outer layers of the tumours, are pathognomonic of HPV infection.

Treatment. Any associated sexually transmitted disease should be excluded, and cervical cytology performed on all patients. Condylomata acuminata are usually treated initially with cytotoxic agents (podophyllin, podophyllotoxin or 5-fluoruracil) but these should be avoided in pregnancy. Destructive procedures (such as the application of trichloracetic acid, cryotherapy or electrocoagulation) may be preferred for recalcitrant condylomas and for papular lesions. Carbon dioxide laser treatment is often chosen by those operators with the necessary skill. Imiquimod, a new immune modulator, can be useful. Subclinical HPV infection of the vulva is probably best left alone.

Molluscum contagiosum

Aetiology. Molluscum contagiosum is a benign viral papular condition, the causative virus being a poxvirus. It replicates in the cytoplasm of infected cells, where it forms large inclusions. Eventually, the nucleus disappears and the cell is entirely occupied by virus – the 'MC body'. The virus has not been replicated *in vitro*.

Clinical features. In children lesions appear on the face and trunk, but in adults they affect the genitals and are sexually transmitted. In women, Molluscum contagiosum appear on the lower abdomen, pubis, labia and adjacent skin. The smallest are rounded pink-grey papules, but as they enlarge they become characteristically umbilicated, 2–5 mm in diameter (Fig. 2.32). They are larger and more numerous in those who are immunosuppressed. Multiple Molluscum contagiosum affecting the face is characteristic of HIV infection. Histologically, there is acanthosis with a central core of Molluscum contagiosum bodies and cell debris.

Diagnosis. The lesions of Molluscum contagiosum may be mistaken for warts or may resemble other papular vulval conditions, but their umbilicated appearance is characteristic. For laboratory diagnosis, the core may be scraped out and examined as a wet preparation for Molluscum contagiosum bodies. Alternatively, biopsy can be performed.

Treatment. The lesions may be destroyed by liquid phenol introduced on a pointed stick, treated by cryotherapy or curetted under local anaesthesia.

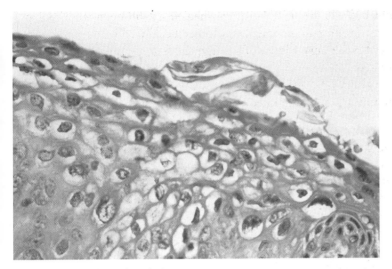

Figure 2.31 Histology of a vulval wart

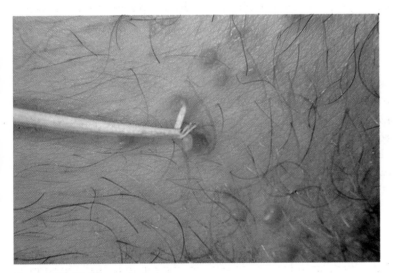

Figure 2.32 Molluscum contagiosum

VULVAL INFECTION AND HIV

Multiple infections of the vulva, particularly by sexually transmitted organisms, are common. In the modern world, HIV is a major health problem, and the virus interacts with vulval infection in two ways. Immunosuppression often leads to a more serious or modified local disease, and vulval lesions, particularly if ulcerated, may facilitate the transmission of HIV. The treatment of vulval infections in women with AIDS may be difficult.

VULVAL INFECTIONS IN CHILDREN

After the menarche, vulval infections are the same as in adults. In pre-pubertal children, the vaginal epithelium is columnar rather than squamous, the pH is 6.5–7.5, and the flora show few lactobacilli. Thus, vaginitis rather than cervicitis is the clinical feature of infections such as gonorrhoea. The ways in which the vulva in children may become infected are:

- transplacental, as in congenital syphilis;
- perinatal, as in herpes and some cases of warts;
- accidental;
- sexual abuse.

Vulvovaginitis

The clinical features include itching, discharge, crusting and erythema, being the same whatever the cause. Potential pathogens – *S. pyogenes, N. gonorrhoeae, H. influenzae, T. vaginalis, C. albicans* and threadworms – must be identified in the laboratory. Vulvovaginal infection with *N. gonorrhoeae* (Fig. 2.33) is likely to be caused by sexual contact: non-venereal 'accidental' gonococcal vulvovaginitis is now rare. *T. vaginalis* infection in children may occur through sexual contact, but perinatal infection from an infected mother is also possible.

Ulcerative conditions

In early congenital syphilis, bullous, papular and papulo-squamous eruptions may affect the vulva during the neonatal period. Condylomata lata appear later, towards the end of the first year.

Infection by HSV types 1 or 2 can occur in children. Perinatal infections are usually maternal, but some type 1 infections may be nosocomial. Genital herpes in older children has the same features as in adults (Fig. 2.34), but the cervix is not affected. An adult's herpetic whitlow may be responsible, but sexual transmission of herpes to abused children is well recognised.

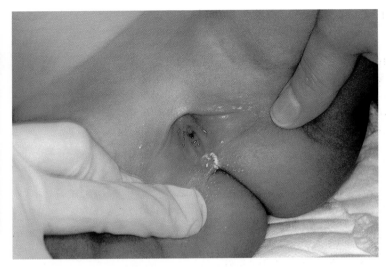

Figure 2.33 Gonococcal vulvitis in a 10-month-old child. Note the discharge at the posterior fourchette and normal hymenal opening.

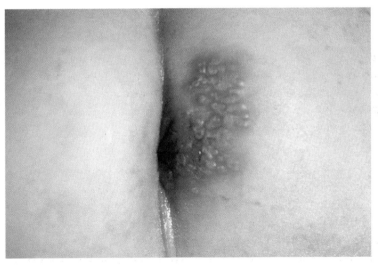

Figure 2.34 Group of vesicles caused by herpes simplex virus type 2 in a child

Papular and condylomatous lesions

Both condylomata acuminata (Fig. 2.35) and papular warts (Figs 2.36 and 2.37) affect the vulva in children. Infection with HPV may be:

- perinatal from a mother with genital warts, the incubation period being up to 11 months;
- via inoculation from cutaneous warts in the child or in an adult;
- the result of sexual abuse.

Pre-menarchal girls with vulval warts are often also infected at internal mucosal sites such as the vagina and anal canal.

Treatment of warts in children

Different treatment modalities have been used in children with good effect but there are no trials of therapy. The spontaneous regression rate is much higher in children than adults, in the order of approximately 50%. For children with warts but without symptoms it may be appropriate to wait for a few weeks. For symptomatic warts, especially if the warts are bleeding and large, surgical removal may be indicated. Podophyllin 10% carefully applied weekly can also be effective. Trichloracetic acid can be used but must be applied carefully and is not suitable for young children. Although podophyllotoxin is not specifically licensed for children, this is purer than podophyllin and is likely to be effective; it can be prescribed on a named-patient basis.

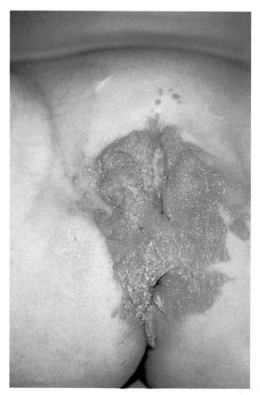

Figure 2.35 Child with condylomata acuminata

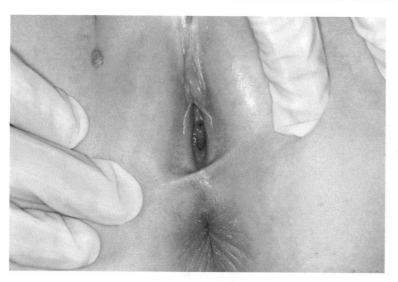

Figure 2.36 Genital warts in a 3 year old girl. Note the normal hymen.

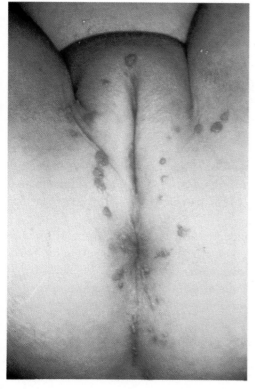

Figure 2.37 Child with papular warts

Molluscum contagiosum in children usually occur at non-genital sites, but vulval lesions can be found (Fig. 2.38). The infection may follow child abuse but is more likely to reach the vulva accidentally from another child. The clinical appearance is similar to that in adults.

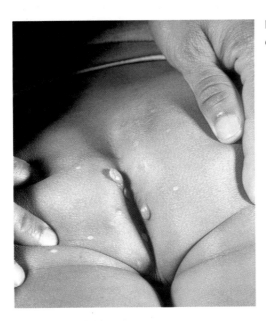

Figure 2.38 Large mollusca contagiosa in a child

PRINCIPLES OF MANAGEMENT OF SEXUALLY TRANSMITTED INFECTIONS

SEXUAL HISTORY-TAKING

In some patients presenting with vulval symptoms, it may be necessary to enquire about their sexual partners. This requires the doctor to have good communication skills and to be sensitive to the needs of the patient, particularly with regard to confidentiality.

During the consultation, one should establish the patient's sexual orientation and the number of sexual partners in the previous month. As some infections, particularly HPV, have a long incubation period, it may be necessary to identify sexual partners over a minimum of 6 months or perhaps longer. It is important to enquire about the use of condoms or other barrier methods of contraception.

Information should be obtained about previous sexually transmitted diseases as well as about previous illness of a medical or surgical nature. In particular, it should be noted whether there is a history of hepatitis.

Many patients have psychosexual difficulties and may present to clinics with physical symptoms. It is an important part of the consultation to elicit psychosexual problems.

The aim of the history and examination is to reach a clinical diagnosis that can be confirmed by initial laboratory tests. Treatment is instigated at the time of the first attendance. The patient is then reviewed with the results of investigations, including confirmation or registration of the findings on initial testing. The advantage of immediate diagnosis and treatment is to reduce the length of infectivity and hence the spread of infection.

PARTNER NOTIFICATION

Formerly called contact tracing, this is an essential part of the management of sexually transmitted infections. If the patient has an infection identified, he or she is asked to inform the sexual partner or partners and to urge them to attend a clinic for a consultation, examination and treatment. This task should be undertaken by staff with training in this aspect of care, that is, health advisors. In the majority of cases, patients are prepared to inform their partners. However, health advisors can, with the permission of the index patient, undertake this task in difficult circumstances.

The importance of contact tracing is not just to prevent reinfection of the index case, but also to identify previous sexual partners who may be infected. The management of patients with sexually transmitted infections concerns not just the individual, but also the public health.

EDUCATION/HEALTH PROMOTION

An increasingly important aspect of all medical care is providing information in an easily understandable form so that patients can make informed decisions about their future behaviour. All patients should be aware of the risk of HIV infection, the protection offered by condoms against the majority of sexually transmitted infections and the importance of avoiding reinfection. Other sexually transmitted infections may act as co-factors for HIV transmission; in developing countries, there are accepted associations between vulval infection and HIV. By the control of other sexually transmitted infections, the prevalence of HIV will be reduced.

Confidentiality, in whatever setting the management of sexually transmitted infections takes place, is of vital importance to encourage those who might be at risk of infection to come forward for screening.

KEY POINTS

1 Remember that more than one vulval infection may be present at any time.

2 Diagnose before carrying out treatment.

3 Contact the patient's partner(s) and refer to a sexually transmitted infection service.

4 Give counselling and advice on safer sex.

5 Preserve a non-judgemental attitude.

6 Supply written information to supplement the consultation.

7 Observe confidentiality.

chapter 3

DERMATOLOGICAL CONDITIONS

INFLAMMATORY DERMATOSES

INTERTRIGO

This is a common erythematous non-specific condition of the flexures, facilitated by obesity, heat and sweating. It often becomes secondarily infected, and when *Candida* is present, small peripheral satellite papules are seen (Fig. 3.1). Predisposing factors should be dealt with as far as possible and the folds kept separated. A combination of topical hydrocortisone and clotrimazole or miconazole is helpful.

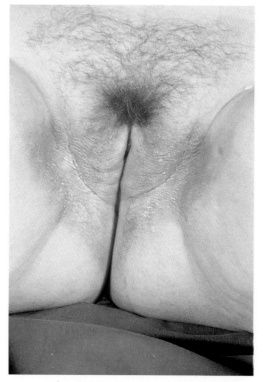

Figure 3.1 Intertrigo; diffuse erythema in the genitocrural folds

ECZEMA, SEBORRHOEIC DERMATITIS AND PSORIASIS

Eczema

Eczema (dermatitis), a primarily epidermal inflammatory process, may be constitutional in origin or caused by irritant or allergic reactions. The keratinised skin is affected, becoming red, scaly and moist (Fig. 3.2). Lichenification is often superimposed because the condition is itchy.

It is important to consider the question of adverse reactions to irritants such as sprays and antiseptics, as well as allergic reactions, where a reaction has developed to something previously tolerated. It seems that allergic reactions, resulting in allergic contact dermatitis, are particularly likely to be found when there is involvement of the perianal area as well as the vulva. The history is of limited value here, and patch testing should be carried out when there is a clinical suspicion and also when the patient has used a variety of medicaments when first seen. It may subsequently have to be repeated if there are unexpected reactions to treatment.

Seborrhoeic dermatitis

The lesions here are diffusely red, and the natal cleft is often involved. Similar patches are often to be found in other areas, for example on the face, behind the ears and on the scalp.

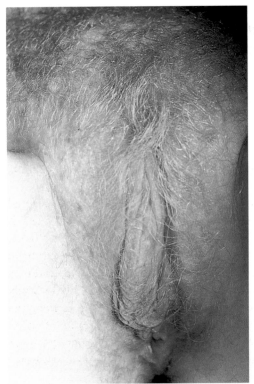

Figure 3.2 Eczema: scaly and moist erythema

Psoriasis

Psoriasis in the genital area is less scaly than it is elsewhere, but the bright erythema and usually sharp outline are helpful in diagnosis (Fig. 3.3), as is the finding of lesions on other parts of the skin, although these are not invariably present.

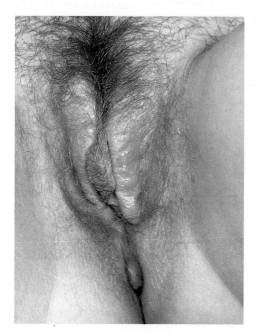

Figure 3.3 Psoriasis: well-defined, bright erythema

Differential diagnosis of eczema, seborrhoeic dermatitis and psoriasis

The differential diagnosis is usually from each other, and this is not often important as the management will be similar. A biopsy will distinguish between eczema and psoriasis, the former showing spongiosis, acanthosis and a perivascular, mainly lymphocytic dermal infiltrate, the latter parakeratosis, acanthosis, an absent granular layer and broad rete ridges with a lymphocytic dermal infiltrate. Seborrhoeic dermatitis has intermediate features. Psoriasis is more resistant to treatment, and when the response is slow, a biopsy will help to confirm the diagnosis and justify trials of other remedies for psoriasis including, on occasion, systemic agents.

There some other conditions, however, that sometimes need to be considered in the differential diagnosis and where management is not the same. Tinea is relatively non-inflammatory but has an active edge, affects the genitocrural area, the inner thighs and often the buttocks, and is unlikely to present a problem unless it has already been misdiagnosed and rendered atypical and florid by corticosteroids (tinea incognito). Erythrasma is non-inflammatory and uniformly brown and scaly. Vulval intraepithelial neoplasia is an important differential diagnosis. Its lesions are pleomorphic and may be red, eroded and extensive. Particularly in the case of eczema, rare conditions such as extramammary Paget's disease, familial benign chronic pemphigus and even glucagonoma syndrome need to be borne in mind.

Glucagonoma syndrome. Glucagonoma syndrome, produced by a glucagon-secreting tumour, usually of the islet cells of the pancreas, is extremely rare, occurring mainly in elderly women. There is a strikingly erythematous circinate, scaly and bullous rash, termed necrolytic migratory erythema, in the anogenital area and elsewhere (Fig. 3.4). The patient is ill and often suffers from diabetes, stomatitis and weight loss. The condition is fatal if untreated. The removal of the tumour and, if applicable, the metastases by hepatic artery embolization can be effective. The administration of octreotide will improve the rash but will not alter the prognosis.

Management of eczema, seborrhoeic dermatitis and psoriasis

The treatment of eczema, psoriasis and seborrhoeic dermatitis consists of potassium permanganate soaks if the condition is acute, followed by bland emollients such as aqueous cream as soap substitutes and as moisturisers, and a corticosteroid, usually with an antibacterial or anti-Candida agent. For mild cases, hydrocortisone with clotrimazole or miconazole will suffice. For others, more potent corticosteroids, for example betamethasone valerate, are needed; psoriasis in particular often initially responds only to these stronger preparations. Dithranol, tar and calcipotriol, used in psoriasis of other parts of the skin, are too irritant to be used on the vulva.

Patch testing may be indicated in some cases of eczema, and in the other conditions too if an adverse effect of local applications is suspected. This will be arranged by the dermatologist. It entails the application to the back of a standard set of substances, which includes corticosteroids, supplemented by those which the patient has been using, and by toilet preparations and cosmetics thought to be of possible relevance. The patches are removed, the results being read after 2 days and re-read after another 2 days. When assessing the results, it is important to decide which are relevant to the clinical picture; nickel allergy, for example, is common but is unlikely to have been responsible for the vulval rash.

LICHENIFICATION AND LICHEN SIMPLEX

Lichenification is a term for the thickening of the skin in response to rubbing and scratching. It is common on a background of eczema or psoriasis. Lichen simplex is used to describe similar changes arising on apparently normal skin. The pattern of the skin is accentuated, and it becomes pale and earthy in colour as well as thick (Fig. 3.5).

A potent or very potent corticosteroid is needed to break the self-perpetuating cycle of itching and scratching. Such an ointment is used nightly until the situation is controlled, usually in a week or two, then less often and eventually just occasionally. Maintenance is thus achieved, the alternative being to switch to a milder preparation for long-term use. Hydroxyzine is often useful at night as a mild anxiolytic. Nail varnish, to which the patient may become allergic, is best avoided, and the nails must be kept short since scratching is often carried out unconsciously while the patient is asleep.

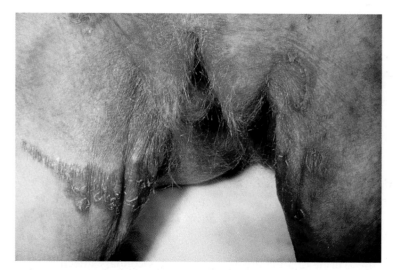

Figure 3.4 Glucagonoma: circinate, scaly and erythematous rash

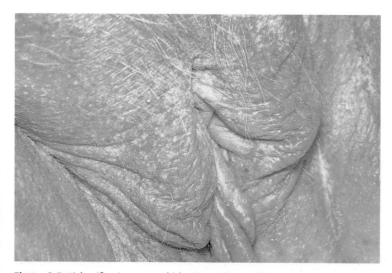

Figure 3.5 Lichenification: gross thickening with magnification of the normal skin markings

The diagnosis of lichenified skin is not difficult. It is, however, important to remember that there may be an underlying eczema or psoriasis. Another condition, albeit a rare one, that may underlie lichenification because it is so intensely itching is Fox–Fordyce disease.

Fox–Fordyce disease

Intensely itchy, skin-coloured papules, mainly affecting the axillae, breasts and pubic area, arise on a basis of obstruction in the apocrine sweat glands.

INFLAMMATORY CONDITIONS IN INFANCY

Napkin rashes

Napkin rashes take three forms. The most common is the irritant type, which is diffuse, largely spares the folds and is related to the effects of wetting, friction, faecal contamination, urine of a pH greater than 8 and secondary infection with Candida and bacteria. Eroded papules sometimes develop. Seborrhoeic napkin rash is not related to seborrhoeic dermatitis in adult life. The rash is diffusely red. Napkin psoriasis again is probably not related to psoriasis in later years, but the rash is psoriasiform with well-defined scaly patches and often lesions elsewhere (Fig. 3.6); in some infants, there is evidence of atopic eczema, but the prognosis in general is good, the eruptions clearing when napkins are no longer worn.

The differential diagnosis includes two rare conditions: acrodermatitis enteropathica and Langerhans cell histiocytosis.

Acrodermatitis enteropathica. Acrodermatitis enteropathica is caused by zinc deficiency, whether as a genetic problem or by way of, for example, prematurity. The rash is fiery and confluent, usually being accompanied by a rash on the face and a loss of hair (Fig. 3.7).

Langerhans cell histiocytosis. In Langerhans cell histiocytosis, the napkin area is involved frequently, as may be other areas of the skin. There is an eruption of yellowish, often purpuric papules; the treatment and prognosis depend upon whether or not there is systemic involvement.

Management of napkin rashes

The management of napkin rashes should be by cleansing with a bland substance such as emulsifying ointment, and the application of a protective substance such as petroleum jelly. Mild corticosteroids, combined with an antifungal or antibacterial agent, are useful. Perhaps the most important measure is frequent changing of the napkin.

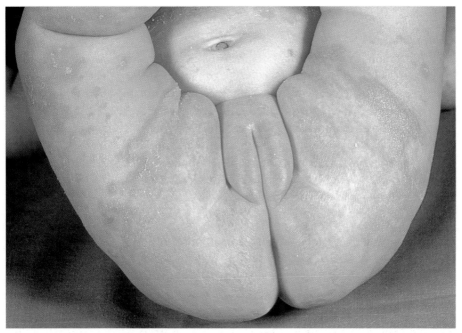

Figure 3.6 Napkin psoriasis: well-defined scaly patches

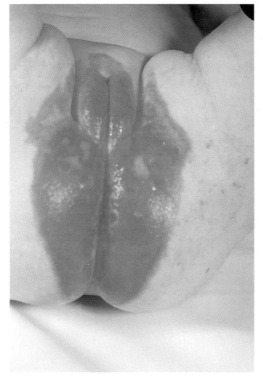

Figure 3.7 Acrodermatitis enteropathica: fiery confluent erythema related to zinc deficiency

OTHER CONDITIONS OF INFANCY AND CHILDHOOD

Labial adhesions

Labial adhesions are not encountered before the age of 2 months and rarely after the age of 2 years. The aetiology is uncertain, but oestrogen deficiency has been postulated. There may remain only a pinhole meatus, situated anteriorly. Scarring related to trauma of any sort, to the bullous disorder cicatricial pemphigoid, and to lichen sclerosus (in which there are, however, usually changes of texture, papules and pallor) are conditions that must be considered in the differential diagnosis, as is the condition of ambiguous genitalia. With labial adhesions, there is a line of demarcation between the clitoral hood and the labia minora, which helps to distinguish them from ambiguous genitalia, although the onset after birth is also important in this respect.

Ambiguous genitalia. Ambiguity of the genitalia arises from different causes, but the phenotype tends to be similar in all cases, usually featuring an enlarged phallus and structures resembling rugose labia majora or scrotal sacs. Early assessment by a specialist gynaecologist or paediatrician is all-important in aiding decisions on surgical intervention and sex of rearing.

Management of labial adhesions

The adhesions often separate spontaneously, or if sealing is leading to urinary problems they can be separated by the mother with bland applications, or with an oestrogen cream for up to two weeks.

LICHEN PLANUS

Lichen planus is of unknown aetiology but is associated with autoimmune disease; it has clinical and histological similarities to lichen sclerosus. Flat-topped, purplish papules on the keratinized skin of the vulva are like those seen in other areas, which may accompany them, and similarly often itch. A whitish network, like that familiar in the mouth, is often seen when the eruption nears or impinges upon mucosal surfaces (Fig. 3.8). The lesions resolve, often leaving postinflammatory hyperpigmentation.

A hypertrophic form has keratotic, warty lesions that can become infected, macerated and painful; its course is chronic (Fig. 3.9).

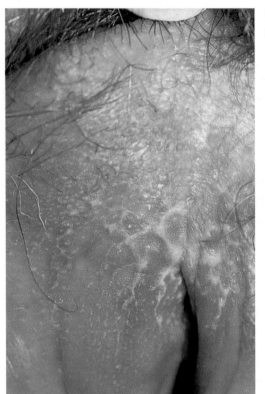

Figure 3.8 Lichen planus: flat-topped papules and whitish reticulation

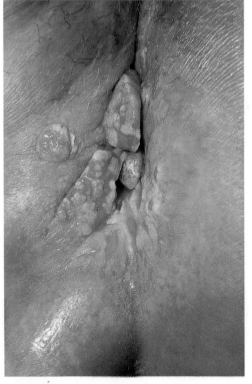

Figure 3.9 Hypertrophic type of lichen planus: eroded nodules and fissuring

A distinctive vulvovaginal-gingival form is very painful and resistant to treatment. All the sites not necessarily being involved contemporaneously (Fig. 3.10). The vaginal wall is eroded, and adhesions may lead to stenosis. All forms of lichen planus may be associated with varying degrees of erosion, atrophy and loss of the normal architecture.

The epidermis has a well-marked granular layer, and there is a dermal band of lymphocytes closely apposed to the epidermis, producing the picture of an interface dermatosis.

The differential diagnosis is mainly from lichen sclerosus, and unless there is vaginal involvement, which does not occur in lichen sclerosus, this distinction can be sometimes almost impossible either clinically or histologically. Other diagnoses to consider are cicatricial pemphigoid and, in the hypertrophic form, malignancy. There is in fact an increased risk of carcinoma in vulval lichen planus, although not, it appears, in the vulvovaginal-gingival syndrome.

Management, except in mild cases, is difficult. Very potent corticosteroids and often oral steroids are required, as occasionally are trials of oral cyclosporin and retinoids. Prednisolone suppositories can be used as pessaries for vaginal lesions. When stenosis is marked, surgical procedures will only be of benefit if carried out in conjunction with the skilled use of dilators and corticosteroids; great harm can otherwise be done, since synechiae promptly seal off the tissue again. For these reasons, as well as because oral problems are often present, management in many cases of lichen planus should be multidisciplinary.

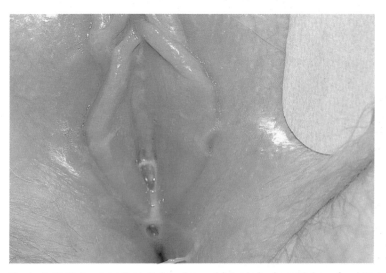

Figure 3.10 Vulvovaginal-gingival syndrome. (a) Eroded vulva with loss of architecture. Note the whitish streaks at the periphery

(b)

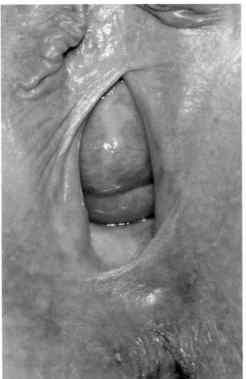

(c)

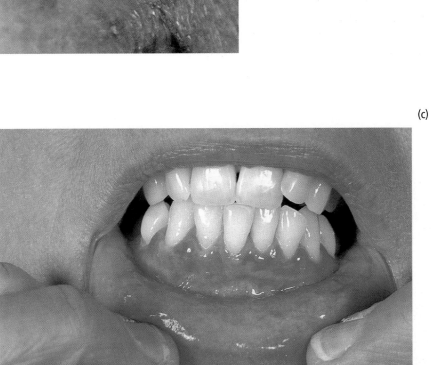

Figure 3.10 Vulvovaginal-gingival syndrome. (b) Erythema of the prolapsed vaginal wall, and loss of vulval architecture. (c) Erosive gingivitis

LICHEN SCLEROSUS

Lichen sclerosus has much in common with lichen planus. There is a marked association with autoimmune disease, most commonly thyroid disorder. Although lichen sclerosus affects all areas of the body, it is most often found in the genital area of women and quite often also in little girls. Its terminology has

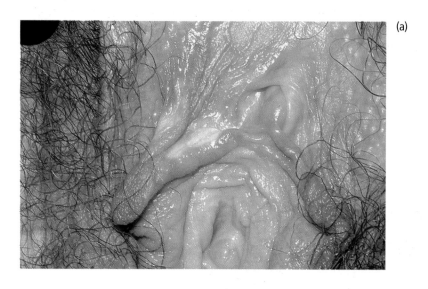

(a)

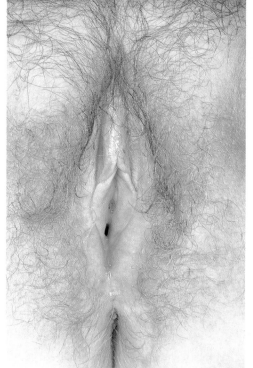

(b)

Figure 3.11 Lichen sclerosus. (a) Small areas of typical pallor and atrophy. (b) Extensive lesions with loss of tissue

been confused in the past but should not be so now; terms such as leukoplakia and dystrophy are meaningless and should never be used.

It is characterized by ivory papules that coalesce into pale plaques, the surface being crinkly and atrophic, often with purpuric markings. The pattern is typically a figure-of-eight, involving the vulva and the perianal area, but small isolated patches are also seen (Fig. 3.11a). The genitocrural folds, all aspects of the labia majora and minora, the clitoris and the introitus may be involved. The clitoris is often sealed over, and in some patients, the contours of the affected parts are obliterated. In severe cases, there is destruction of all the tissue (Fig. 3.11b and c). Itching is usually marked but may also be entirely absent.

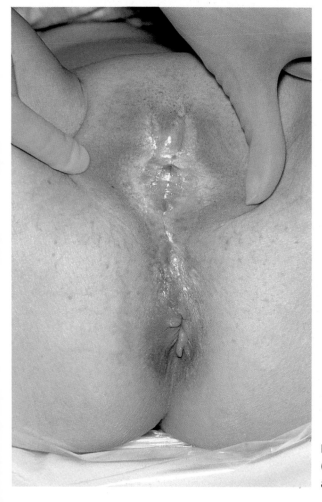

Figure 3.11 Lichen sclerosus. (c) Obliteration of the contours and sealing over

The epidermis may be thin, or hyperkeratotic with pointed and elongated rete pegs, and a band of lymphocytes is separated from the epidermis by a characteristic zone of hyalinization, although this may not always be obvious in vulval specimens.

The differential diagnosis is mainly from lichen planus, cicatricial pemphigoid and vitiligo, the skin in the latter condition being white but without any change in texture.

The patient should be given adequate information on her condition and made fully aware of how to use the treatment advised. There is no place for topical oestrogen or testosterone. A very potent topical corticosteroid, for example clobetasol propionate 0.05 per cent ointment, in a reducing régime such that not more than 30 g are used in 3 months, is dramatically effective and appears to be safe. It should be coupled with bland emollients. Indefinite maintenance with small amounts is satisfactory; where destruction has not occurred, the tissues may eventually look normal. Very rarely, the condition is resistant to this treatment, and topical or even systemic retinoids may be tried.

There is undoubtedly an increased chance of carcinoma in lichen sclerosus. Neoplasia can arise in non-symptomatic cases, and it is not yet known whether or not effective treatment will modify the risk. The formation of hyperkeratotic plaques or erosions that do not respond to treatment should arouse suspicions of malignancy and calls for biopsy. In the absence of malignancy, there is no indication for surgery, with the exception of a careful vaginoplasty where introital stenosis is causing symptoms, or sometimes a meticulous unsealing of tissue around the clitoris. Tests of thyroid function will often be indicated.

Lichen sclerosus in girls

The appearance is essentially similar to that in adults, and treatment is the same, although 30 G of the very potent corticosteroid should last for at least 6 months rather than 3. Used judiciously, it will arrest the progress and prevent the destruction that may occur (Fig. 3.12a and b). Vitiligo and bullous disease are the main differential diagnoses, but sexual abuse has to be borne in mind. Lichen sclerosus may be mistaken for abuse, especially when infected (Fig. 3.12c) or haemorrhagic (Fig. 3.12d), but the two may co-exist. The condition improves at puberty, although complete resolution is probably rare and it may recur later. It may be that effective treatment will modify prognosis.

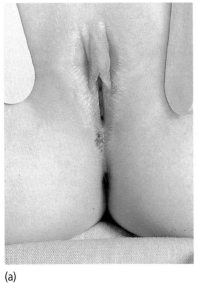

(a)

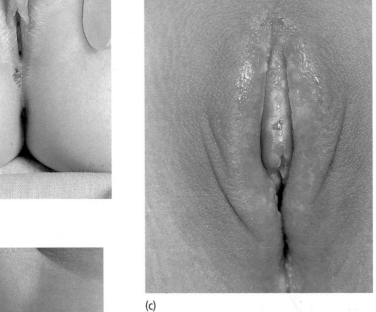

(c)

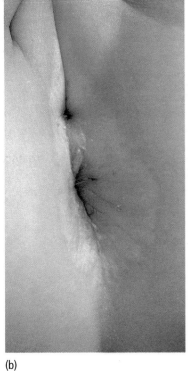

(b)

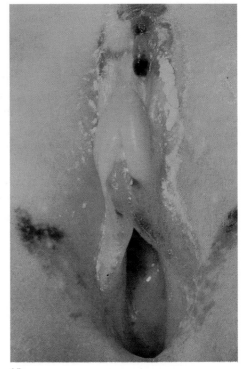

(d)

Figure 3.12 Lichen sclerosus in a child.
(a) With marked pallor. (b) Perianal
involvement. (c) Secondary infection.
(d) Haemorrhagic lesions

BULLOUS (BLISTERING) DISORDERS

Bullae at this site often rupture and appear as erosions. The disorders are of varying aetiology.

FAMILIAL BENIGN CHRONIC PEMPHIGUS (HAILEY–HAILEY DISEASE)

This is inherited as an autosomal dominant condition. Moist scaly patches affect the flexures; they are precipitated or worsened by infection or contact allergy (Fig. 3.13). The histology is diagnostic, showing extensive acantholysis. Immunofluorescence is negative. Histologically, and to some extent clinically, Darier's disease is a differential diagnosis to be considered. More importantly, however, the condition is easily mistaken for an intertrigo or eczema.

Treatment with topical corticosteroids and topical and oral anti-infective agents is effective.

STEVENS–JOHNSON SYNDROME

This syndrome is a form of erythema multiforme with mucosal involvement. It may be related to drugs or infection, notably with herpes simplex virus, or be idiopathic. Genital, oral and ocular involvement is usual, and there may or may not be lesions, usually acral and of typical iris pattern, on the skin (Fig. 3.14).

Severe cases should be nursed in a burns unit. The use of systemic steroids is controversial. Cyclosporin has been used with benefit. Topical and oral antibiotics should be used only in accordance with culture findings, since resistant organisms can be a problem. Scarring of the vulva and vagina may ensue.

TOXIC EPIDERMAL NECROLYSIS AND STAPHYLOCOCCAL SCALDED SKIN SYNDROME

These conditions are clinically but not histologically identical, the bullae being subepidermal in the former and intraepidermal in the latter. The former is idiopathic or drug induced; the latter, most often seen in children, is caused by a staphylococcal exotoxin, usually of phage type 2. The clinical picture is of widespread, intensely painful peeling areas, with mucosal involvement, and the patient is very ill.

The treatment of toxic epidermal necrolysis is as for Stevens–Johnson syndrome, that of staphylococcal scalded skin syndrome being with antibiotics. Again, scarring may be a sequel.

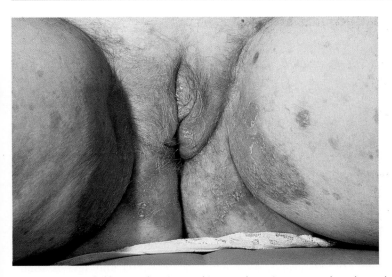

Figure 3.13 Familial benign chronic pemphigus: scaly, moist areas on the vulva and genitocrural area

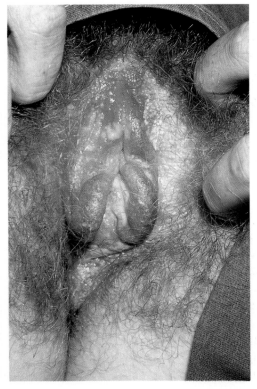

Figure 3.14 Stevens–Johnson syndrome: an eroded bulla on the mucosal surface

IMMUNOBULLOUS DISORDERS

In these conditions, antibodies develop against the epidermal cells or basement membrane. A blister is the result of an interaction between the antibodies and the target cells, which are those concerned in adhesion between the cells. The level of the bulla depends on the nature of the target cell. Indirect immunofluorescence (IMF) may demonstrate circulating antibodies in the blood, and direct IMF deposits of immunoglobulin at the relevant sites. Clinically based terminology is giving way to a more exact characterization in terms of the target cells, and changes in nomenclature are consequently to be expected.

Pemphigus vulgaris

Pemphigus is rare. Extragenital lesions are usually to be found.

The vulval lesions are painful and eroded, and vaginal extension may occur (Fig. 3.15). There is no scarring.

The bullae are intraepidermal, with much acantholysis and IgG is found between the epidermal cells.

Linear IgA disease of children (formerly chronic bullous disease of childhood) and adults

In childhood, there is a particular predilection for the genital area, clusters of bullae being seen on keratinized skin, for example of the pubic area (Fig. 3.16). There are tense subepidermal blisters, and IMF shows a band of IgA at the basement membrane zone. The condition tends to improve at puberty, but scarring may remain.

Bullous pemphigoid and cicatricial pemphigoid

Both these eruptions are rare. Tense bullae affect the genital area and, particularly in the case of cicatricial pemphigoid, may also affect the vaginal, ocular and oral mucosa. Both conditions show subepidermal bullae with a deposition of IgG at the basement membrane zone, but they can be distinguished clinically by the scarring and loss of normal architecture associated with cicatricial pemphigoid.

Differential diagnosis of immunobullous disease

The conditions mainly need to be differentiated from each other, and much depends on histology and immunofluorescence. Cicatricial pemphigoid can resemble lichen planus and lichen sclerosus.

Management of the autoimmune bullous diseases

Because of the frequent involvement of other mucosal surfaces and the serious disability found in many patients, management in the care of a multidisciplinary team is desirable. Except for the mildest cases, which can be controlled by very potent topical corticosteroids, systemic treatment is required. This may be sulphapyridine or dapsone in linear IgA disease of children, but in other conditions may include steroids, immunosuppressive agents such as azathioprine and cyclosporin, drugs used empirically, for example minocycline and nicotinamide, and measures such as plasmaphoresis.

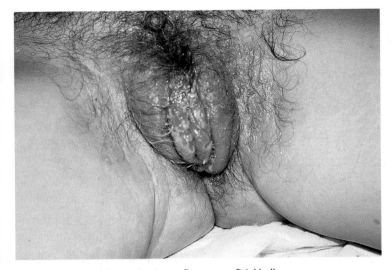

Figure 3.15 Pemphigus vulgaris: confluent superficial bullae

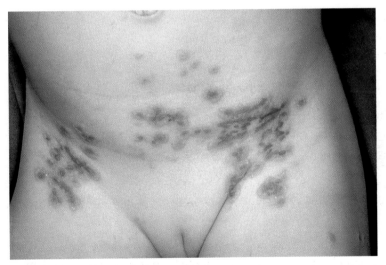

Figure 3.16 Linear IgA disease in a child: clusters of bullae

CONDITIONS CHARACTERIZED BY PIGMENTARY CHANGES

Pigmentation in neoplasms is noted elsewhere.

PIGMENTATION RELATED TO HAEMOSIDERIN

Haemosiderin deposits are common in prolapsed tissue, in caruncles and in association with lichen planus and lichen sclerosus. Their colour is a reddish brown.

Zoon's plasma cell vulvitis

A striking deposition of haemosiderin is a feature characterising the appearance of plasma cell vulvitis, which is, however, of uncertain status. The changes are described mainly on the labia minora and in the vestibule. Many examples could be classified as lichen planus or lichen sclerosus, but a small idiopathic and distinctive group, with certain other histological characteristics, may remain.

With regard to treatment, some cases improve with topical flamazine or clindamycin.

PIGMENTATION RELATED TO MELANIN

Hyperpigmentation

Here one should distinguish between post-inflammatory changes, which are more common in dark-skinned subjects and in relation to some conditions, notably lichen planus (Fig. 3.17), and those related to an intrinsically pigmented eruption. With respect to the latter, melanosis, fixed drug eruption, acanthosis nigricans and pseudo-acanthosis nigricans deserve mention.

Melanosis

Melanosis denotes macular pigmented patches that are usually multiple and symmetrical (Fig. 3.18), sometimes being accompanied by similar oral changes. They are persistent but apparently benign, showing histologically basal hypermelanosis and an increased number of normal melanocytes. It is essential to biopsy such lesions, the differential diagnosis including lentigines, moles, seborrhoeic warts and, above all, pigmented vulval intraepithelial neoplasia.

Fixed drug eruption

A fixed drug eruption recurs at the same site after the ingestion of the drug in question (for example tetracycline or phenolphthalein) as a tumid dusky plaque that may blister and then resolves to leave a deeply pigmented area.

Acanthosis nigricans

Acanthosis nigricans is a rare condition, which when it occurs in children is benign, but which in adults is virtually always associated with malignancy, the site of which must be sought. All cases are thought to be fundamentally linked to insulin resistance. Darkening of the skin, especially in the flexures and genital

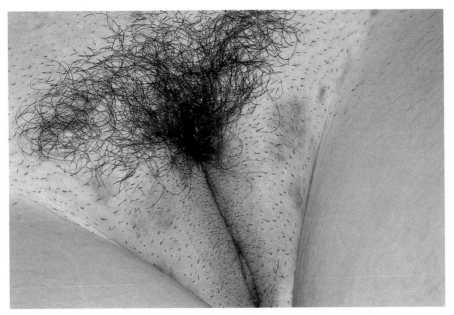

Figure 3.17 Post-inflammatory pigmentation: brown areas following the resolution of lichen planus

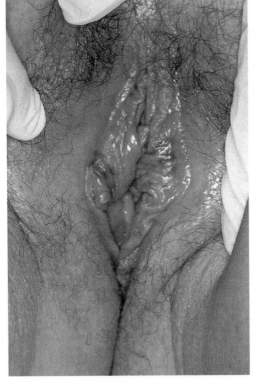

Figure 3.18 Melanosis: multiple symmetrical brown-black macules

area, evolves to become velvety and then warty; the mouth is affected and the palms thickened. Treatment is of no avail. The clinical picture is somewhat similar to that of Darier's disease, which is, however, histologically distinctive.

Darier's disease

In this rare condition, inherited through an autosomal dominant gene, there are extensive, rather dark warty papules that, in the flexures, become macerated. However, the long history in Darier's disease and its distinctive histology, showing extensive acantholysis, suffice to make the distinction from acanthosis nigricans possible. Histologically, Darier's disease is more likely to be confused with familial benign chronic pemphigus (Hailey–Hailey disease).

Pseudoacanthosis nigricans

Pseudoacanthosis nigricans is associated with obesity, especially in the dark skinned. The changes are confined to the flexures, which are dark and velvety or warty, often with small tags. These features improve if weight is lost.

Hypopigmentation

Here again, one sees post-inflammatory pigmentary changes, particularly in dark-skinned individuals (Fig. 3.19), and conditions that are intrinsically hypo-pigmented or depigmented, such as lichen sclerosus and vitiligo.

Vitiligo

Vitiligo is completely white except sometimes for a hyperpigmented rim or some patchy pigmentation if there is a tendency to repigment round a hair follicle; it tends to be symmetrical (Fig. 3.20). Lichen sclerosus has some change of texture, but this can be minimal. Moreover, lichen sclerosus and vitiligo not infrequently occur together, and a distinction can be difficult. Post-inflammatory changes, particularly in a black skin and if there is scarring, can closely mimic vitiligo. There is no effective treatment for genital vitiligo.

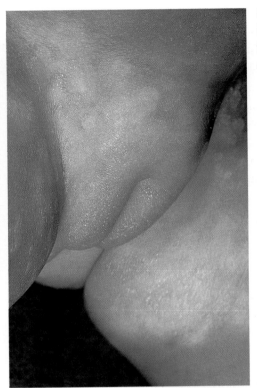

Figure 3.19 Post-inflammatory hypopigmentation: diffuse pale areas following a napkin rash in a dark-skinned child

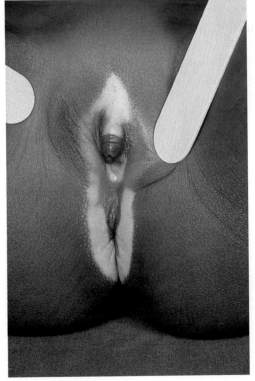

Figure 3.20 Vitiligo: symmetrically disposed depigmented areas

CONDITIONS CHARACTERIZED BY ULCERS

The manifold causes of vulval ulcers are listed in Chapter 1, infective ulcers are described in Chapter 2 and malignant ones in Chapter 5. Some of the non-infective conditions are discussed here.

BEHÇET'S SYNDROME

This syndrome of probable viral aetiology is rare, particularly in women, and should be diagnosed only in strict accordance with agreed criteria, that is: recurrent oral ulceration plus two of the following – recurrent genital ulcers, eye lesions, cutaneous lesions or a positive pathergy test. A period of observation may be required before the diagnosis is certain. The ulcers are painful, chronic and tend to scar (Fig. 3.21).

APHTHOUS ULCERS

The major form of oral aphthous ulcers (Fig 3.22a) is sometimes accompanied by similar vulval ulcers (Fig. 3.22b). The aetiology is unknown, there sometimes being a genetic background. The ulcers are again painful and recurrent.

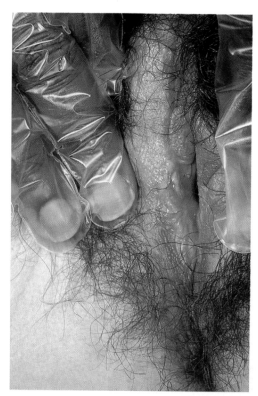

Figure 3.21 Behçet's syndrome: solitary ulcer

OTHER ULCERS

Acute, solitary or sparse non-recurrent ulcers sometimes appear in adolescent girls, often with fever and malaise. Some are probably associated with viral infections, particularly infective mononucleosis.

DIFFERENTIAL DIAGNOSIS AND MANAGEMENT OF ULCERS

The differential diagnosis is from the infective ulcers, especially recurrent herpes simplex, from eroded bullae in bullous disorders, occasionally from malignant ulcers and more rarely from unusual lesions such as artefacts or drug eruptions. The recurrent nature of ulcers in Behçet's syndrome and aphthous ulceration, and the general clinical picture, is important, since their histology is non-specific.

In Behçet's syndrome, the milder examples will respond to topical corticosteroid and tetracycline preparations such as triamcinolone (10 mg/mL) 5 mL mixed with 95 mL tetracycline syrup, but others will need systemic therapies, which include colchicine, azathioprine and thalidomide. Topical symptomatic treatment is effective in the other forms of ulcer.

(a)

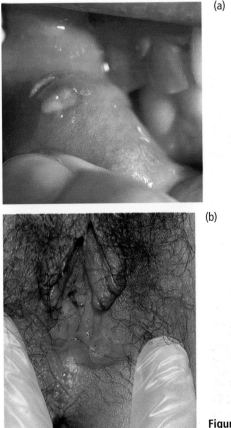

(b)

Figure 3.22 (a) Aphthous ulcer of mouth.
(b) Aphthous ulcer of vulva

SCARRING

Causes of scarring have been listed elsewhere (*see* Ch. 1), and several, for example lichen sclerosus, cicatricial pemphigoid and Behçet's syndrome, have been described in this chapter. There is one important condition that should, however, be noted here: hidradenitis suppurativa.

HIDRADENITIS SUPPURATIVA

Hidradenitis suppurativa, at one time thought to be a disease of the apocrine glands, is now attributed to changes in the epithelium of the hair follicle. It begins after puberty, often affecting the axillae and breasts as well as the groins and anogenital area. Milder cases show recurrent inflammatory lesions with painful swellings and abscesses, leading to typical bridged scars with comedones (Fig. 3.23). In severe cases, there is swelling, destruction of tissue, sinuses and gross scarring. Neoplasia has been reported as a rare complication.

The main differential diagnosis is from Crohn's disease. In the latter, scarring is not as prominent, but swelling and sinuses are often found; bowel signs may not be present, nor may the typical granulomatous histology. In hidradenitis, the presence of lesions elsewhere, the bridged scars, are helpful.

Antiandrogens are sometimes of help, but long-term antibiotics are probably more effective. Retinoids have been used with variable results. Surgery is of assistance in dealing with small localized areas. In severe cases, there is considerable morbidity, with a disturbance of general health, and surgery is the best choice. At this stage, it often needs to be extensive, invoving grafting or healing by secondary intention.

(a)

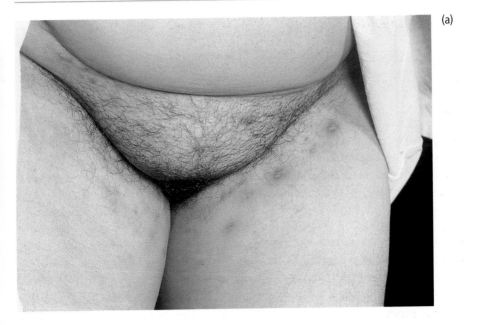

(b)

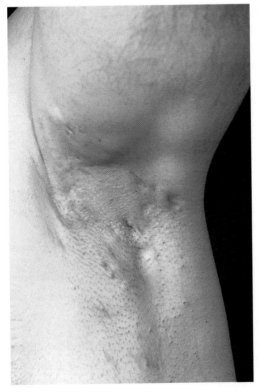

Figure 3.23 Hidradenitis suppurativa.
(a) Extensive scarring in the groin.
(b) Bridged scars and comedones in the
axilla

OEDEMA

Causes of vulval oedema are given in Chapter 1. Some will be enlarged upon in this section.

Vulval tissue is lax and readily becomes oedematous, for example in cardiac failure. Local reactions are more often responsible, and swelling is marked in angioedema, Candida infections and acute contact dermatitis. The acute contact urticaria type 1 reaction set up in susceptible subjects by contact with latex in condoms, caps and examination gloves is more serious and may produce anaphylaxis and death. Similar but usually less severe reactions occasionally arise in the form of allergy to seminal fluid.

LYMPHOEDEMA

This may be primary, related to congenital lymphatic hypoplasia, or secondary. Important causes of the latter type, apart from infections such as lymphogranuloma venereum, are obstruction from malignant deposits, the effects of surgery after inguinal lymphadenectomy, the effects of radiotherapy in that area, sometimes hidradenitis suppurativa and Crohn's disease (Fig. 3.24).

Crohn's disease

The changes of Crohn's disease in the anogenital area may antedate the onset or detection of bowel disease and need not be anatomically continuous with the bowel. Sinuses and ulcers, fistulae and abscesses, mingle with inflamed perianal tags on a background of marked oedema (Fig. 3.25). The oedema may be unilateral or generalized. Granulomatous cheilitis or changes in the mouth referred to as cobblestone-like are often present. The histology may show granulomatous changes suggestive of Crohn's disease but may also show only non-specific oedema and lymphatic dilatation.

As noted above, the main differential diagnosis is hidradenitis suppurativa, in which scarring is more marked and oedema less so, but idiopathic lymphoedema must also be borne in mind.

Course and management of lymphoedema

The tissue becomes indurated and is subject to recurrent attacks of cellulitis, which in turn increases the swelling. These can be prevented by long-term penicillin V or erythromycin administration. Small lymphangiectases appear as little vesicles along the dependent edges and are sometimes mistaken for warts. Laser treatment can control these effectively.

TRAUMA

Trauma in relation to sexual abuse and radiation is considered in Chapter 6.

SURGICAL AND ARTEFACTUAL TRAUMA

While the vulva heals well, punch biopsy scars for example usually leaving no trace, many patients will have scars that the examining doctor may find difficult to assign. Such are the scars of episiotomies, operations on Bartholin's gland,

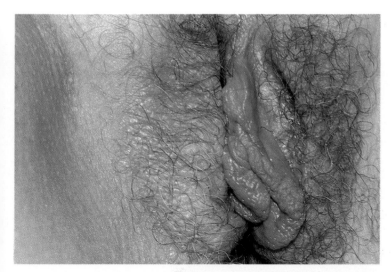

Figure 3.24 Lymphoedema on a background of Crohn's disease. Note the lymphangiectases

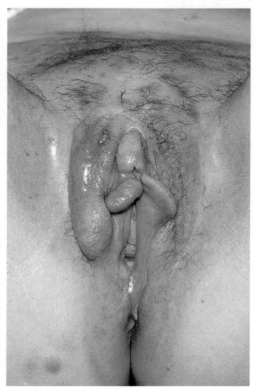

Figure 3.25 Crohn's disease: oedema, swelling, indurated areas and sinuses

Fenton's operations and more major surgery for vulval intraepithelial neoplasia and carcinoma. It is useful to become familiar with these changes. Artefactual injury is rare but should be considered in any unusual presentation. One important albeit rare condition – pyoderma gangrenosum – may, however, affect the vulva and mimic an artefact.

Although usually seen on a background of ulcerative colitis or rheumatoid arthritis, *pyoderma gangrenosum* may occur in association with myeloproliferative disorders and in otherwise healthy women. The clinical appearance is striking: a large chronic ulcer, often of bizarre shape with a dusky overhanging edge, gradually enlarges. Much depends upon clinical recognition since the histology is non-specific. Control is usually achieved with steroids, dapsone or minocycline.

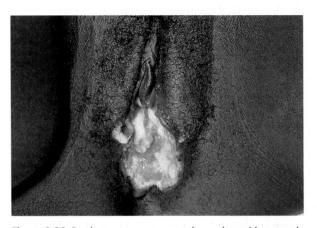

Figure 3.26 Pyoderma gangrenosum; a large ulcer with an overhanging edge

KEY POINTS

1 In patients with inflammatory dermatoses, always be aware of the possibility of superimposed irritant and allergic reactions if the response to treatment is not straightforward.

2 In suspected immunobullous disease, biopsy and immunofluorescence studies will be needed.

3 In lichen planus and lichen sclerosus, remember the increased risk of malignancy and biopsy any suspicious areas.

4 A loss of vulval architecture usually suggests a diagnosis of cicatricial pemphigoid, lichen planus or lichen sclerosus.

5 Common things commonly occur, but rare ones sometimes do too and should be borne in mind.

chapter 4

VULVODYNIA

DEFINITION

Vulvodynia is defined as chronic soreness, burning or pain, as opposed to itching (pruritus). If it is not clear in the history which is predominantly being complained of, the patient should be asked whether she has the wish to scratch; in vulvodynia the answer will be no, in itching yes. The pain is often clearly accounted for by a chronic infection or an inflammatory dermatosis. When it is not accounted for thus, or when it persists after treatment and the resolution of physical signs, the patient has one of two conditions – vulval vestibulitis or dysaesthetic vulvodynia – between which there may be some overlap (Table 4.1).

AETIOLOGY

These two disorders are now considered to be essentially problems of chronic pain, and our understanding of them has gradually evolved over the 25 or so years in which they have been recognized. The concept of a chronic pain problem has proved a good working hypothesis and is supported by the response to appropriate treatment. A working explanation is that some trigger factor sets off inappropriate impulses in pain fibres, which in turn sensitize the dorsal horn cells so that afferent impulses of light touch in myelinated fibres are misinterpreted as

Table 4.1 Vulvodynia (vulval burning, pain or soreness). After the exclusion of any symptoms attributable to infection and dermatoses, the following should be considered

	Symptoms	Abnormal physical signs
Vulval vestibulitis	Specifically related to attempted vaginal entry. Acutely tender on point pressure	Variable and minimal; sometimes patchy erythema
Dysaesthetic vulvodynia	Independent of attempted vaginal entry. Often constant. No tenderness on point pressure	None
Overlap group	Variable. Often a combination of those in the above groups	Usually none

pain. There is 'cross-talk' between these afferents and efferent sympathetic fibres, which themselves keep the process going by acting upon the myelin of the afferent fibres. Moreover, central mechanisms become involved. The outcome is a state in which pain becomes the response to light touch and is abnormally heightened and prolonged.

This condition will be new territory for many of the doctors consulting this book. A lack of experience in dealing with it can to some extent contribute to its perpetuation and even worsening. In many situations the best course will be to refer the patient to a setting, usually a specialized vulval clinic, where management, although often not easy for either the doctor or the patient, is likely to be optimal. Conversely, the doctor who first recognizes the condition can do much good by giving it a name, reassuring the patient at the same time that it is recognized and that there are no implications of infection or malignancy.

VULVAL VESTIBULITIS

Vestibulitis is encountered mainly in younger women. It is defined as the complex of pain on attempted vaginal entry, that is, sexual intercourse or tampon insertion, and acute tenderness on vestibular point pressure, bearing in mind that some degree of the latter is common in asymptomatic women. There may or may not be some patchy erythema, which, if present, is histologically non-specific and of no diagnostic significance. Vestibular papillomatosis may be seen but is irrelevant. There has often been a sudden onset with a trigger factor such as childbirth, surgery, an infection or some psychologically stressful event. Patients subsequently tend to be treated, or to self-treat, for candidal infection without any supporting evidence. Psychosexual problems, either primary or secondary, are common.

Safe symptomatic treatment consists of soap substitutes such as aqueous cream, and 5 per cent lignocaine ointment, perhaps with hydroxyzine as a mild anxiolytic at night. Most women settle well on this regime, but some develop more persistent pain and merge into the category of dysaesthetic vulvodynia; they should then be treated as such. Vestibulectomy has its proponents, but follow-up studies are not entirely persuasive.

DYSAESTHETIC VULVODYNIA

Dysaesthetic vulvodynia is encountered mainly in post-menopausal women. It may complicate other conditions such as lichen sclerosus or lichen planus. The pain is unprovoked, that is, unrelated to intercourse, is constant and is not accompanied by any physical signs or tenderness on pressure. It may be treated with lignocaine 5 per cent ointment or, more often, with low-dose amitriptyline, for example 10 mg at night increasing by 10 mg weekly until the pain is controlled, up to a maximum of about 70 mg, being continued for weeks or months and repeated as necessary. Some patients do not tolerate amitryptiline well so other drugs may be tried; the selective serotonin re-uptake inhibitors are, however, less effective than the tricyclic group. When management is difficult, help should be sought from a pain clinic. Biofeedback and cognitive therapy may be helpful.

In both vestibulitis and dysaesthetic vulvodynia, the situation as we understand it at present should be explained to the patient and her anxieties explored as far as is practicable. Psychosexual counselling may be called for in some cases.

THE FUTURE

At the International Society for the Study of Vulvovaginal Disease Congress in 1999, an amended classification of vulvodynia was proposed and is likely to be adopted (Table 4.2).

Table 4.2 Vulval Dysthaesia (Vulvodynia)

1. Generalized

2. Localized: for example
    Vestibulodynia
    Clitorodynia

KEY POINTS
1 Distinguish between the symptoms of itching and pain.
2 If soreness and pain are the complaint, look for a cause such as an inflammatory dermatosis.
3 If there is no apparent cause, prepare to consider the condition as dysaesthetic vulvodynia or vestibulitis.
4 If progress is unsatisfactory, think sooner rather than later about referral to a specialized clinic.

chapter 5

NON-NEOPLASTIC
SWELLINGS AND
NEOPLASMS

Unless the diagnosis of a lesion as benign and without indication for treatment is absolutely certain, all lumps should be biopsied or removed for examination.

NON-NEOPLASTIC SWELLINGS

As well as cysts, these comprise ectopic tissue, for example endometrioma; or varicosities, urethral caruncle (Fig. 5.1) or prolapse of the urethral mucosa, the latter usually in children or the elderly; cystocoele, rectocoele and procidentia. Deposits of endometrial tissue are usually attributable to implantation following surgery; they are bluish-red and undergo cyclical variation. Varicosities (Fig. 5.2) are not as a rule of serious import, being transient in pregnancy or occasionally persistent in older women, but marked examples or a sudden onset are an indication for investigation since they may be caused by pelvic congestion or obstruction.

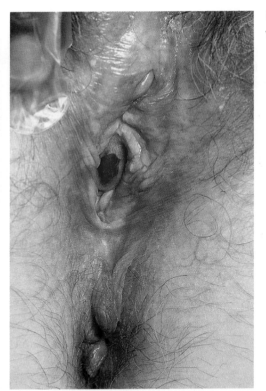

Figure 5.1 Urethral caruncle: a cherry-red, vascular nodule

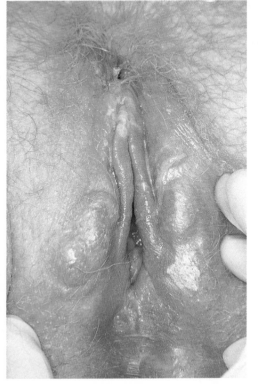

Figure 5.2 Varicosities in a pregnant woman

CYSTS

Cysts may be developmental, when they are often congenital; epidermoid; or related to sebaceous gland blockage (Fig. 5.3). The latter are easily recognized by their yellowish colour; they may be single, sparse or strikingly multiple. Patients often request treatment, and simple evacuation and cautery, or destruction with a Hyfrecator (*see* Ch. 7), is effective. The position and histology will enable the others to be categorized. Cysts of Bartholin's gland duct are initially acute and painful, and their site is diagnostic.

NEOPLASMS

NON-EPITHELIAL TUMOURS

Benign

Benign non-epithelial tumours include fibromas, which appear as firm, smooth nodules usually on the labia, and neurofibromas, which may be solitary or part of a generalized neurofibromatosis type 2 syndrome.

Haemangiomas of the cavernous type (strawberry marks) will not be seen after childhood since their natural course is to resolve spontaneously. Angiokeratomas are common in older women and are found mainly on the labia majora (Fig. 5.4). They present as small papules, dark red or almost black, which are punctate or rather larger, and may be single or multiple. The darkness of solitary angiokeratomas may lead to a mistaken suspicion of melanoma. Small multiple papules can be difficult to distinguish from the purpuric speckling of lichen sclerosus. Treatment, if desired, is by laser, excision or cautery.

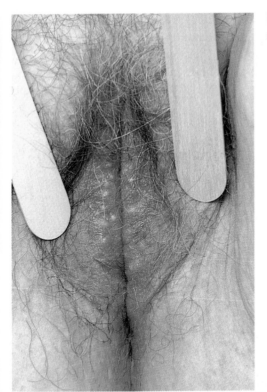

Figure 5.3 Yellowish nodules related to sebaceous gland blockage

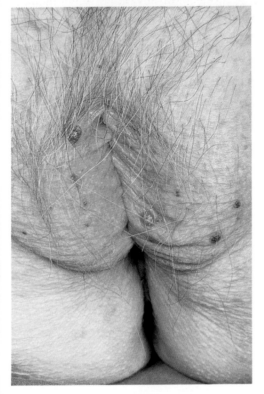

Figure 5.4 Angiokeratomas: dark red lesions with a scaly summit in an elderly woman

Lymphangiomas may not be truly neoplastic. Lymphangioma circumscriptum has small frogspawn-like vesicles that often contain blood and, because of the connection with deep lymphatic cisterns, local destruction may result in recurrence (Fig. 5.5). A similar appearance may result from lymphatic obstruction, as for example in Crohn's disease, following surgery to the lymph glands or after radiotherapy.

Granular cell tumours arise from Schwann cells and the vulva is a site of predilection, although they are uncommon. Neurofibromas and fibromas must be considered in the differential diagnosis; the yellowish colour of granular cell tumours can be helpful.

Malignant

Malignant neoplasms in this category, such as sarcomas and lymphomas, are very rare.

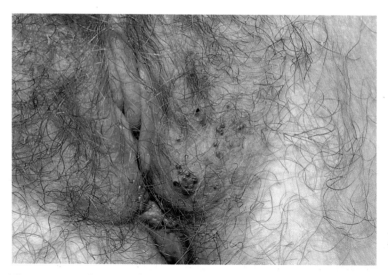

Figure 5.5 Lymphangioma: frogspawn-like vesicles (often blood filled, as here) in a unilateral distribution

EPITHELIAL NEOPLASMS

Benign

These include genital warts, skin tags and seborrhoeic warts. Diagnosis is not as a rule difficult, and they are all simple to remove.

Malignant

Vulval intraepithelial neoplasia. Vulval intraepithelial neoplasia (VIN) does not present as a tumour and may mimic benign dermatoses. As usually employed, the term 'vulval intraepithelial neoplasia' alone will be taken to mean squamous intraepithelial neoplasia (Table 5.1).

Table 5.1   Vulval intraepithelial neoplasia: classification of the International Society for the Study of Vulvovaginal Disease

SQUAMOUS TYPE		
VIN1	Undifferentiated type	Mild dysplasia
VIN2	Undifferentiated type	Moderate dysplasia
VIN3	Undifferentiated type	Severe dysplasia, carcinoma *in situ*
VIN3	Differentiated type	Carcinoma *in situ* (atypicality confined to parabasal area)
NON-SQUAMOUS TYPE		
EXTRAMAMMARY PAGET'S DISEASE		

Undifferentiated squamous VIN is classified as being of full thickness (VIN3) or of a lesser grade (VIN1 and VIN2). It is customary to refer only to VIN3 when discussing its potential for development into a squamous carcinoma. The somewhat confusingly termed VIN3 of differentiated type is, however, a different matter, even though its manifestations are confined to the lower part of the epidermis; it is sometimes seen in lichen sclerosus and probably has some malignant potential in those circumstances.

VIN3 of undifferentiated type, particularly in younger women, is closely related to the human papillomavirus (HPV), especially types 16, 18 and 31. It has become much more common in recent years. It has a strikingly pleomorphic appearance, and the lesions may be red, white, pigmented, warty, moist or eroded as well as solitary or multiple (Figs. 5.6 and 5.7). The papular and pigmented versions are sometimes referred to as Bowenoid papulosis, a clinical term that is not associated with any histological distinction. In older women, solitary patches, with a less clear relationship to HPV infection, are more often found. All parts of the vulva, perineum and perianal area may be affected, either in whole or in part. When the condition is diagnosed, it is important to check all the lower genital tract and anal canal, and to ensure that these areas are kept under regular supervision. Lesions in these other parts, particularly the cervix, are common and often of greater seriousness for the patient in terms of progression to invasive carcinoma. Such change is most likely in those who are immunosuppressed, including the elderly and smokers.

The treatment of this form of VIN3 is difficult (*see* Ch. 7). In a young, non-immunosuppressed patient with no symptoms, there is a case for observation as long as biopsies of any suspicious area are carried out promptly. Local excision is best for small lesions but can lead to a degree of mutilation when used for widespread ones. Laser destruction has drawbacks in that it does not reveal the histology and will be inadequate, short of scarring, for extension down the hair follicles. Cryotherapy and 5-fluorouracil have their disadvantages and limitations, and photodynamic therapy is currently being explored. Even after the excision of clinically apparent disease, recurrence or the appearance of new areas is common, and the risk of progression to invasive carcinoma is not eliminated. Whenever foci of invasion are found, the treatment is as for squamous carcinoma.

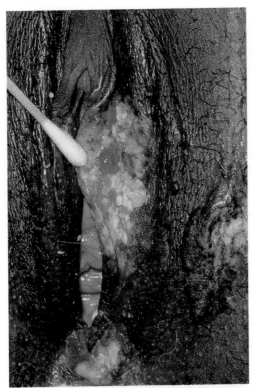

Figure 5.6 Vulval intraepithelial neoplasia: reddish white patches

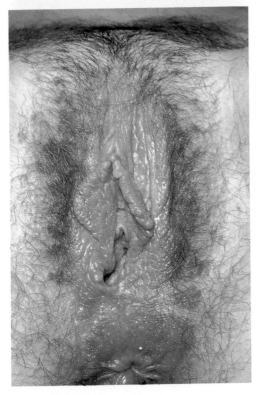

Figure 5.7 Vulval intraepithelial neoplasia: pigmented warty areas

Non-squamous VIN. Non-squamous VIN is extramammary Paget's disease. It is rare, and is eczematoid in appearance, so diagnosis is often delayed. This eczematoid appearance is accounted for by the presence of the typical Paget cells within the epidermis. The moist, red, scaly patches may affect any part of the vulva, perineum and perianal area, and may be localized or widespread (Fig. 5.8). The changes tend to extend beyond the clinical margins.

The initial treatment is usually by excision since there is in some cases an underlying adenocarcinoma. Small recurrences can be treated with 5-fluorouracil cream or other modalities. There is an increased risk of associated neoplasms elsewhere, particularly in the anogenital area or breast, and judicious screening should be carried out.

Squamous cell carcinoma. Squamous cell carcinomas are the most common malignant vulval tumours. They present as hard, often ulcerated and bleeding lesions, or may be discovered not as a lump but histologically, as a focus of invasion seen on biopsy of an area of VIN. They occur at any site but most often on the labia (Fig. 5.9). They arise upon undifferentiated VIN3, lichen sclerosus, occasionally lichen planus and less often apparently normal skin. There is a bimodal pattern of incidence. Younger women generally have carcinomas associated with HPV and undifferentiated VIN3. Older women tend to have carcinomas arising upon lichen sclerosus or lichen planus, sometimes associated with epithelial cell hyperplasia or VIN3 of the differentiated type, or neoplasms arising on no known pre-existing skin condition. In this older group, the role of the HPV is debated but certainly less apparent.

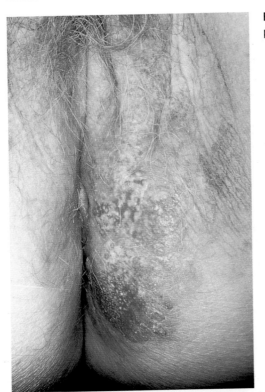

Figure 5.8 Eczematoid appearance of Paget's disease

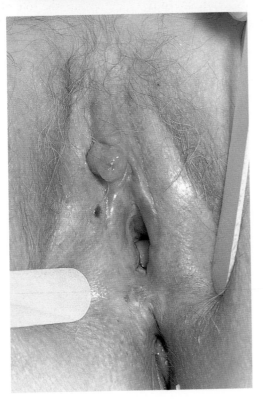

Figure 5.9 Squamous cell carcinoma, here arising on lichen sclerosus

It is important to ensure that the size of the tumour and the depth of the invasion are measured accurately as treatment depends upon these. Individualization for early tumours, avoiding extensive mutilating surgery, is now known to be practicable. The current approach is based upon criteria of staging (Tables 5.2 and 5.3).

Table 5.2 International Federation of Obstetrics and Gynecology: Staging criteria for squamous carcinoma of the vulva (1994)

Stage 1: lesions 2 cm. or less confined to the vulva or perineum; no lymph node metastases.

Stage 1a: lesions 2 cm. or less confined to the vulva or perineum with stromal invasion no greater than 1.0 mm (measured from the epithelial-stromal junction of the adjacent most superficial dermal papilla to the deepest point of invasion); no lymph node metastases.

Stage 1b: lesions 2 cm. or less confined to the vulva or perineum with stromal invasion greater than 1.0 mm; no lymph node metastases.

Stage II: tumour confined to the vulva and/or perineum more than 2 cm in the greatest dimension with no nodal metastases.

Stage III: tumour of any size arising on the vulva and/or perineum with (a) adjacent spread to the lower urethra and/or the vagina or anus and/or (b) unilateral regional lymph node metastases.

Stage IVa: tumour invading any of the following: upper urethra, bladder mucosa; rectal mucosa; pelvic bone and/or bilateral regional lymph node metastases.

Stage IVb: any distant metastases including pelvic lymph nodes.

Reproduced with permission from Shepherd J.S., UK representative, Gynaecological Cancer Committee, International Federation of Gynecology and Obstetrics, Cervical and vulval cancer; changes in FIGO definitions of staging. *British Journal of Obstetrics and Gynaecology*, 1996; **103**: 405–6.

Table 5.3 Individualization of the treatment of squamous carcinoma of the vulva: criteria for depth of invasion, size and site

Stage Ia: wide local excision

Stage Ib: lateral lesion; wide local excision plus ipsilateral lymphadenectomy, with contralateral lymphadenectomy if the glands are found to be positive

Stage Ib: central lesion; radical vulvectomy and bilateral lymphadenectomy

Stages II, III and IV: radical vulvectomy and bilateral lymphadenectomy

If the lesion is greater than 4 cm in diameter, pelvic lymphadenectomy should be considered

Adapted with permission from Hacker, N.F. and Van der Velden, J., Conservative management of early vulvar cancer. *Cancer*, 1993; **71**: 1673–7.

Verrucous carcinoma. The rare verrucous carcinoma (giant condyloma of Buschke and Loewenstein) is of dramatic appearance, being large and warty. It is histologically benign but clinically malignant, burrowing relentlessly. Local excision is effective.

Adnexal neoplasms. The only benign adnexal neoplasms likely to be encountered are the syringoma, derived from eccrine sweat glands and presenting as small skin-coloured papules, with or without similar lesions elsewhere, and the hidradenoma, probably derived from apocrine glands and presenting as skin-coloured nodules that are as a rule solitary and may on occasion become eroded. Syringomas can be excised or destroyed by, for example, laser treatment. Hidradenomas are excised.

Basal cell carcinomas are not uncommon malignant adnexal neoplasms. They extend locally, often more than is clinically apparent, but rarely metastasize. They appear as firm nodules or ulcers, sometimes pigmented (Fig. 5.10), and are often of long duration. They should be excised; micrographically controlled surgery may reduce the risk of recurrence.

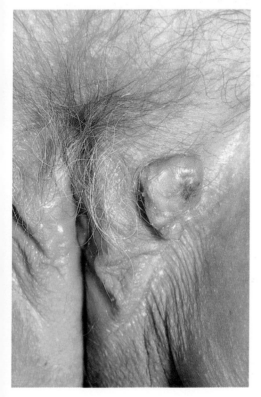

Figure 5.10 Basal cell carcinoma: pigmented nodule

Metastatic carcinoma. Metastatic carcinoma at the vulva is usually from a primary tumour of the cervix, endometrium, vagina, ovary, urethra, kidney, breast, rectum or lung. The deposits are firm, single or multiple, cutaneous or subcutaneous masses (Fig. 5.11).

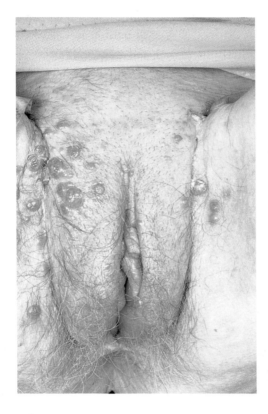

Figure 5.11 Metastatic carcinoma, from a primary ovarian tumour

Melanocytic neoplasms. Benign moles are common and may be junctional, compound or intradermal. Rarer types peculiar to the vulva may also be seen. Excision is sometimes advisable, even if there is nothing to suggest malignancy, since the site often makes it difficult for the patient to keep the lesion under observation. The most important differential diagnosis is pigmented VIN.

Malignant melanoma may arise *de novo* or on a pre-existing mole. It is usually but not invariably pigmented, and is often not diagnosed until it has become a bleeding and ulcerated mass (Fig. 5.12). The prognosis is determined, as at other sites, by the depth of invasion. Surgery should be guided by this, and wide local excision, as with melanomas elsewhere on the skin, does not worsen the prognosis as compared with radical vulvectomy.

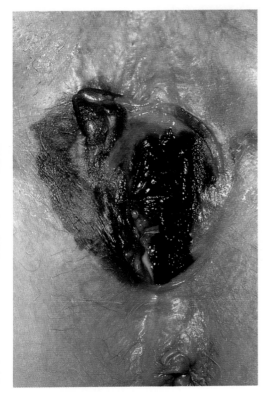

Figure 5.12 Malignant melanoma: ulcerated pigmented plaque

NEOPLASMS OF THE URETHRA AND BARTHOLIN'S GLAND

Neoplasms of the urethra and Bartholin's gland are occasionally encountered and may be of squamous, adenocarcinomatous or transitional cell type.

KEY POINTS

1 Remember that VIN can closely mimic a dermatosis.
2 When VIN is found, be sure to check the vagina and cervix for similar changes.
3 Always be aware of the possibility of a focus of invasive cancer in VIN.
4 When a patch of 'eczema' does not respond to treatment, think of Paget's disease and biopsy it.
5 The non-gynaecologist must be aware of when to refer the patient to a gynaecologist, and of the modalities of treatment currently thought to be the best.

chapter 6

TRAUMA AND ABUSE

Trauma and abuse to the genital area may result in physical signs that need to be distinguished from those of other vulval pathology.

Trauma may be iatrogenic, accidental, self-inflicted, a result of unusual practices such as female genital mutilation (FGM), or caused by sexual assault. In the majority of cases of sexual assault, in both children and adults, there are no physical signs.

The most appropriate clinicians to investigate suspected abuse are the designated doctors for child sexual abuse present in each district. There are usually child protection teams with multidisciplinary membership, and it is recommended that possibly abused children are referred to such an experienced team.

HISTORY-TAKING AND EXAMINATION

Patients may volunteer information about the nature of their injury. Another important factor to explore is the psychological state of the patient, particularly in relation to self-inflicted injuries.

If there is any suspicion of abuse, accurate documentation is vital. If specimens are taken for forensic purposes a 'chain of evidence' must be demonstrable for the evidence to be admissable in court (Table 6.1).

Table 6.1 Laboratory chain of evidence form

CLINICAL DEPARTMENT

Lab. No:	Date received:			Time received:	
Patient's details:				Specimen type:	
Doctor's name:				Specimen taken by:	
Signature:				*Signature:*	
Specimen delivered to lab by:					
Signature:					

Microbiology department	NAME	SIGNATURE	DATE	TIME
Received by MLSO:				
Doctor check at receipt:				
Consultant check of final report:				
Organisms to save:				

There may be a distortion of the normal anatomy in some circumstances, for example FGM, which makes the diagnosis of other vulval conditions more difficult. In addition, abuse may coexist with other pathologies.

USE OF THE COLPOSCOPE

A colposcope provides a light source and magnification. It also has the advantage of an in-built measuring device. This gives an accurate measurement of the hymenal orifice in children, and more accurate information on the extent of injury in adults. An attached camera is easily used, photography often being the best means by which to record visual aspects of the clinical situation. Photographs may also be employed to obtain second opinions and as evidence in court. Permission must be sought when taking medical photographs, and documentation of when and by whom they were taken is required.

Care is needed in the interpretation of colposcopic findings as there is uncertainty surrounding the incidence of minor variations in the normal population. The colposcope is unlikely to reveal significant findings of abuse that would otherwise go undetected by an experienced examiner, but it may increase the detection of minor signs by up to 10 per cent.

IATROGENIC TRAUMA

POST-LASER TREATMENT

Secondary adhesions may occur after the lasering of lesions of the labia minora and vestibule, and synechiae may form (Fig. 6.1). The partly fused labia may tear during sexual intercourse.

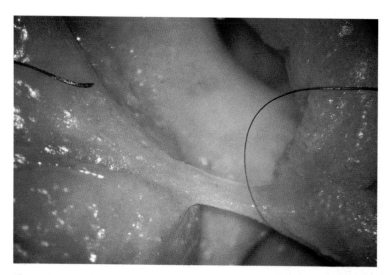

Figure 6.1 Synechiae post-laser treatment

POST-RADIATION INJURY

Radiation damage has been a complication of earlier methods of radiotherapy used for carcinoma of the vulva and following radiation for inguinal lymphadenopathy (Fig. 6.2a). Radio-dermatitis is occasionally encountered in patients with lichen sclerosus whose intractable pruritus was treated with radiation in pre-topical corticosteroid days (Fig. 6.2b).

Radiation damage predisposes to malignancy, and patients at risk should be advised accordingly.

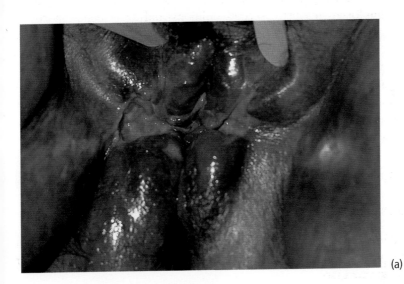

(a)

(b)

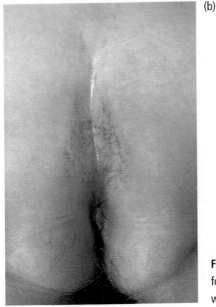

Figure 6.2 (a) Radionecrosis; deep ulceration following radiotherapy. (b) Radiodermatitis in a patient who had radiotherapy for pruritus of lichen sclerosus.

ACCIDENTAL INJURY

Accidental injury is often caused by straddle injuries and stretching, which result in tearing, and penetrating injuries caused by sharp objects may also occur. Injury may in due course lead to abscesses, keloids, cysts, neuromas or calculi. In women of child-bearing years, there is sometimes an increased risk of further problems in subsequent labours.

OBSTETRIC TRAUMA

The passage of the fetal head through the birth canal may frequently result in tearing of the vulva, usually through its weakest point, that is, the fourchette. Modern obstetric practice seeks to divert the tearing forces with an episiotomy incision to the right or left of the midline. However, recent suggestions that healing from a tear is more satisfactory than that from an episiotomy has led to more tears and fewer episiotomies. A primary tear involves the perineum, a second-degree tear extends to the muscles surrounding the anal sphincter and a third-degree tear involves the sphincter, leading to faecal incontinence.

There may be copious haemorrhage at delivery when pregnancy-induced varices are present in the labia majora. Haematomas may complicate delivery and can be life threatening. Vulval trauma may be exacerbated after FGM practised in African countries has rendered the outlet reduced and scarred. The unskilled use of obstetric forceps, especially those used in rotating the vertex, may also damage the vulva during delivery.

Careful suturing following all forms of obstetric vulval trauma often results in satisfactory healing. Third-degree tears must always be repaired by skilled and experienced gynaecologists.

Episiotomy scars (Fig. 6.3)
Granulation tissue or ulceration may occur in the episiotomy scars, giving rise to superficial dyspareunia. Refashioning of the episiotomy scar may help.

POST-COITAL FISSURES

At first intercourse, hymenal tears are to be expected, usually occurring posterolaterally. These fissures heal rapidly in a few days, leaving behind a pale scarred area that may tear again on subsequent intercourse. During consensual sexual intercourse, fissuring may also occur at the posterior fourchette, underlying skin disorders, for example lichen sclerosus, predisposing to fissuring at this site. Areas of scarring can fissure during examination, particularly when there is tension on the hymenal ring.

Patients present with localized burning of the vulva triggered by micturition or intercourse. Symptoms tend to be recurrent, occurring with each intercourse. Bland emollients may help, but surgical treatment may sometimes be considered.

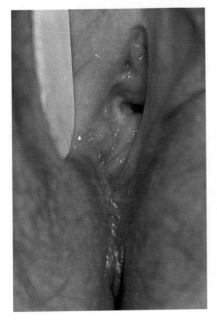

Figure 6.3 Tender nodules of granulation tissue in an episiotomy scar eight weeks after delivery

SELF-INFLICTED INJURY

The genital area is a recognized site of self-inflicted injury, particularly in disturbed adolescents.

Foreign bodies may be inserted into the vagina, resulting in some trauma. In children, these cause vulvovaginitis in about 30 per cent of cases and may also disrupt the hymen, with recurrent bleeding in up to 50 per cent; this can be difficult to differentiate from child sexual abuse. Children who have been sexually abused may draw attention to their genitals by inserting foreign bodies. If a foreign body is suspected in a child, examination under anaesthetic is appropriate.

Trauma in the form of scratching or minimal accidental injury may lead to purpura and frank bleeding in lichen sclerosus. In other itchy vulval conditions, scratch marks, thickening and fissuring (Fig. 6.4) may be evident.

FEMALE GENITAL MUTILATION

This is uncommonly seen in Western Europe but is the cultural norm in some parts of Africa, particularly Somalia, Ethiopia and the Sudan. It is also carried out along the southern part of the Arab peninsula and the Persian Gulf. In Indonesia and Malaysia, it is practised in a less drastic form, although no surveys have been made. In the UK, FGM was prohibited in 1985 after the passing of legislation. In most other European countries as well as Canada, Australia, New Zealand and most recently the USA, the practice has been criminalized.

TYPES OF GENITAL MUTILATION

There are three types of operation. Clitoridectomy is the least mutilating and involves the removal of the prepuce of the clitoris. This is the only procedure that can correctly be called circumcision.

The most extreme form of FGM is infibulation (or pharaonic circumcision), which involves the removal of the clitoris and labia minora, and the partial removal of the labia majora, followed by a method of fastening or sewing together what remains (Fig. 6.5). In the Sudan and Somalia, thorns are used to hold the two bleeding sides of the vulva together, or a paste of gum arabic, sugar and egg is used to close the wound. In West Africa, closure is achieved by tying the girl's legs together in a crossed position immediately after the operation and immobilizing her for several weeks until the wound has closed. Infibulation is performed to guarantee virginity; the smaller the opening, the higher the bride's price.

In the intermediate form of operation, called 'excision' the clitoris is wholly or partially removed, together with part of the labia minora, the cut edges being sutured together to leave a small opening.

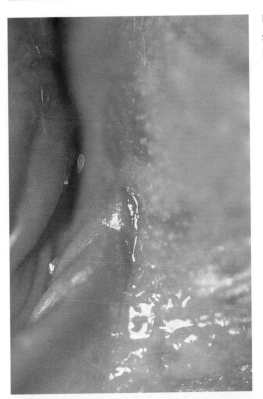

Figure 6.4 Fissuring on the labia minora secondary to scratching during candidal infection

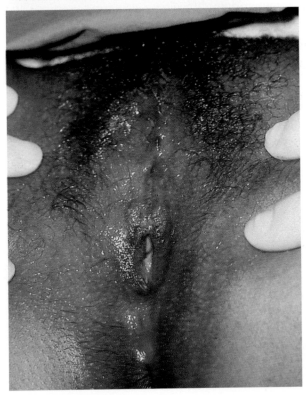

Figure 6.5 Female genital mutilation: infibulation. (Reproduced with permission of the Royal College of Obstetricians and Gynaecologists from *The Diplomate*, 1998; **5**(2)

All these operations are performed on the ground under primitive conditions and without anaesthetic. Since the same implements are used on all the girls in a group operation, the transmission of infection is inevitable. In the case of fatalities, neither the operator nor the operation is blamed: it is claimed that an evil spirit is responsible or that the ritual was not performed properly, or the girl may be held to be at fault because she had sexual intercourse before being operated upon.

IMMEDIATE COMPLICATIONS

Severe pain, shock, haemorrhage, tetanus, sepsis, urinary retention, ulceration of the genital region and injury to the adjacent tissue are all encountered.

LONG-TERM COMPLICATIONS

Cysts, abcesses, keloid scar formation, damage to the uretha resulting in urinary incontinence, dyspareunia and sexual dysfunction may follow.

Infibulation can cause severe scar formation, difficulties in urination and during menstruation, and recurrent bladder and urinary tract infection. Cuts have to be made to allow sexual intercourse.

PREGNANCY – ASSOCIATED PROBLEMS

Complications include fetal monitoring difficulties, caesarean section and obstructed labour leading to fetal death and vesicovaginal fistulae. During vaginal delivery, there may be extensive perineal tearing and damage to the urethra.

PSYCHOSEXUAL AND PSYCHOLOGICAL HEALTH

Many girls and women are traumatized by their experience but, with no acceptable means of expressing their fears, suffer in silence. Women are subject to anxiety, depression, chronic irritability and sexual problems.

Dyspareunia or apareunia may occur, sometimes requiring surgery for normal intercourse to take place.

LEGAL ISSUES

Over the past three decades, ethnic groups who practice FGM have immigrated to Britain, mainly as refugees. The main groups are from Eritrea, Ethiopia, Somalia and the Yemen, where it has been estimated that over 80 per cent of women have had an operation, usually infibulation. There is evidence that the operation is being performed illegally in Britain by medically qualified or unqualified practitioners. In Britain, the procedure is usually performed between the ages of 7 and 9 years. Alternatively, children may be sent abroad for a 'holiday' to have it carried out.

Under the Prohibition of Female Circumcision Act 1985, it is an offence to 'excise, infibulate or otherwise mutilate the whole or any part of the labia majora or minora or clitoris of another person' and 'to aid, abet or procure the performance by another person of any of the these acts on that other person's own body'. A person found guilty of an offence is liable to a fine or to imprisonment for up to 5 years if convicted.

There are specialist clinics run in some central London hospitals providing gynaecological and obstetric care for women who have undergone FGM. Clinics may also offer deinfibulation.

SEXUAL ABUSE

ADULTS

Sexual assault is a relatively common occurrence, with reports of up to 10 per cent of adult women being abused at some point in their lives.

The severity of injuries is extremely variable (Fig. 6.6). The documentation of other physical injuries is paramount in identifying supporting evidence for an assault. However, the majority of women who have been raped – up to 70 per cent – show no evidence of trauma. Injuries are more likely to be present in virgins or with violent abusers. Forensic medical examiners must be conversant with the definitions of injuries (Table 6.2), and physicians and gynaecologists dealing with possibly abused patients should also be aware of these.

CHILDREN

It is important to understand the development of genitalia from the neonatal status to pubescence. At birth, the presence of maternal oestrogen produces transient vulval and hymenal engorgement, the vulval epithelium subsequently thinning. The vestibular skin is normally redder in young girls than in adults. The hymenal orifice may be crescentic, annular or fimbriated. In normal children, the hymenal margin is smooth with no disruption of the blood vessels (Fig. 6.7). Septal remants and septate hymen are rare but normal findings.

Table 6.2 Definition of injuries

Abrasion	supericial injury where the skin or mucous membrane has been scraped away
Blistering	intact fluid-filled vesicles
Bruising	superficial injury, without a break of the skin, resulting in a haematoma or contusion
Erythema	reddening of the skin that blanches when pressed
Incision	a clean, straight-edged wound from a sharp instrument
Induration	hardening of the tissue
Laceration	a torn, ragged-edged wound from a sharp instrument
Swelling	transient enlargement of the tissues
Ulcer	a defect or excavation of the skin surface resulting from the sloughing (or casting off) of inflammatory, necrotic tissue
Fissure	a break in the continuity of the skin or mucous membrane. It can be acute or chronic, single or multiple
Bleeding	and the presence of **scars** should also be noted

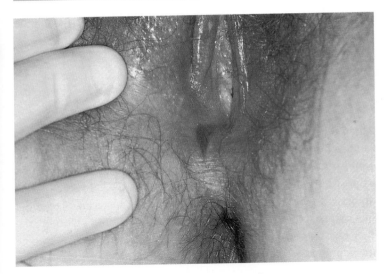

Figure 6.6 A healing laceration 2 weeks after an assault

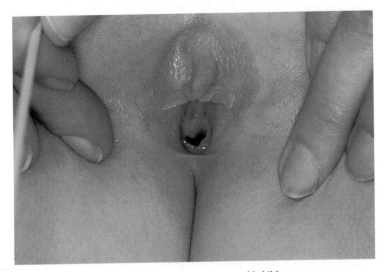

Figure 6.7 A normal crescentric hymen in a 4-year-old child

With the approach of puberty, endogenous oestrogen is produced, causing the epithelium to thicken. These differences influence the microbiological flora of the genital tract.

The normal anus is closed by the action of the internal and external anal sphincters. The presence of normal perianal folds depends upon an intact external sphincter mechanism.

Examination of abused children

The recommended position for the genital examination of most girls is supine and in the frog-legged position with the hips flexed and the soles of the feet touching. This is the easiest position for examination with the colposcope.

Gentle traction between the thumb and index finger at the posterior edge of the labia shows the hymen and posterior fourchette (Fig. 6.8). During the examination, other signs of sexual abuse should be recorded (Table 6.3). The perianal areas are examined with the child lying in the left lateral position or the prone knee–elbow position. The latter may also be used to examine the hymen, particularly if there is difficulty in visualization of the posterior rim.

To examine for reflex anal dilatation, the buttocks are gently separated using the palms of both hands to apply some traction to the anus. The anus should be observed for approximately 30 seconds to see whether the anal canal opens. Should both the internal and external anal sphincters relax, the anal canal slowly opens up, revealing a clear view into the rectum; this is called reflex anal dilation (Fig. 6.9). The perianal region is inspected for signs of inflammation, injury,

Table 6.3 Vulvovaginal signs of sexual abuse

DIAGNOSTIC OF PENETRATION
Laceration or scars extending into the vaginal wall
Attenuation of the hymen with a loss of hymenal tissue

SUPPORTIVE OF PENETRATION
Enlarged hymenal opening
Notch associated with scarring
Localized erythema and oedema
Scarring of the posterior fourchette

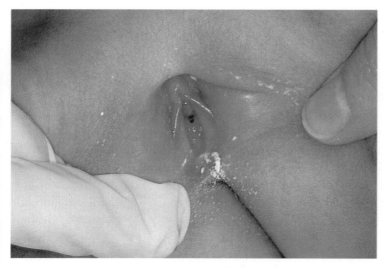

Figure 6.8 Light traction to reveal the posterior fourchette and hymen in a 10-month-old girl. Note the discharge caused by *Neisseria gonorrhoeae*

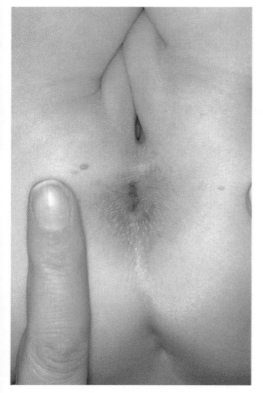

Figure 6.9 Reflex anal dilatation in a child. Note also the genital warts

venous congestion and skin abnormality. The veins and symmetry of the radiating skin folds of the anal verge should be noted (Fig. 6.10). Digital examination is usually unnecessary. Abnormal anal signs in relation to abuse are listed in Table 6.4.

Screening for infection

Most sexually transmitted organisms have been reported in children. Scant data exist on their incidence and prevalence, although in most series the latter is less than 6 per cent. The transmission of infections following abuse must be differentiated from the acquisition of infection by vertical or other means (Table 6.5). Factors affecting the acquisition of sexually transmitted organisms include the prevalence of sexually transmitted organisms in the abusing population, the type of abuse, the mode of delivery, the sexual maturity of the child and the time of examination in relation to the abuse.

Sampling techniques for infection must be appropriate for the sexual maturity of the child. Vulvovaginal, rather than cervical, cultures are required for identification of *Neisseria gonorrhoeae* and *Chlamydia trachomatis* as both these organisms exist on the mucosa of the infected pre-pubertal vagina and vulva. Samples may be obtained either by using swabs or from vaginal washings. The former should be taken with cotton-tipped swabs, moistened if necessary with sterile water, either trans-hymenally or from the posterior fourchette.

Table 6.4   Anal signs of sexual abuse

DIAGNOSTIC OF PENETRATION
Evidence of force or penetrating trauma, e.g. a laceration or healed scar extending beyond the anal mucosa

SUPPORTIVE OF PENETRATION
Acute changes
       Erythema
       Swelling
       Bruising
       Fissures
       Venous congestion

Chronic changes
       Thickening of the anal verge skin
       Increased elasticity
       Reduction of sphincter tone

Anal laxity

Reflex anal dilation (RAD) >2 cm

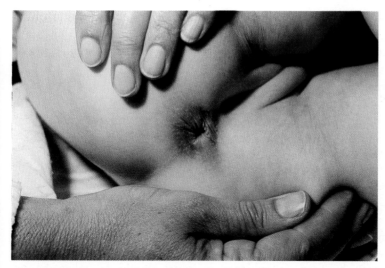

Figure 6.10 Perianal venous engorgement and surrounding bruising of the anus in a sexually abused 3-year-old girl

Table 6.5   Modes of transmission of sexually transmitted organisms in children

Route	Disease/organism
In utero	HIV, syphilis, HPV
Perinatal	*Chlamydia trachomatis*
	Neisseria gonorrhoeae
	HSV
	HPV
	HIV
Direct contact	
Non-sexual/autoinoculation	HPV, HSV
Transmission from fomites	?*Trichomonas vaginalis*
Sexual assault	All sexually transmitted organisms

HPV = human papillomavirus; HSV = herpes simplex virus.

Samples from the anal canal should be taken for the identification of *N. gonorrhoeae* and *C. trachomatis* if anal abuse is suspected.

Particular attention must be paid to using the diagnostic technique that is appropriate for evidence to be admissible in court (*see* below).

Most children allow the taking of specimens without trouble on the first occasion. It is important to ensure that all the investigations (Table 6.6) are undertaken then, as repeat testing has proved more problematic.

Vulval appearances such as labial adhesions and congenital abnormalities may be confused with changes caused by abuse, as may lichen sclerosus, especially if it is infected or haemorrhagic. It should be emphasized, however, that these conditions and abuse may co-exist (Fig. 6.11).

For further information on vulval infections in children, see Ch. 2.

FORENSIC MEDICAL SAMPLES

Samples that may be used as evidence in court should be taken by an appropriately trained doctor working as a forensic medical examiner in the company of a police officer.

Forensic samples fall into two categories: evidential, and control samples for comparison. The evidential trace materials are of two types; one occurs as loose debris or particles, and the other as stains. Particulate debris can be removed with forceps or swabs. Stains can be swabbed with plain cotton swabs, moistened with distilled or tap water (not saline) if dry.

Useful evidence can be obtained from unwashed clothing, bedding, carpets and items used in the assault. These can be examined for blood, semen, saliva, vaginal fluid, faeces, etc. These secretions may also be present on the skin and in the anal canal or vagina.

For samples to be admissible in court, a 'chain of evidence' must be followed. This means that each sample should be labelled with the name of the patient, the date it was taken, the type of sample and the person taking the sample. When these are passed from the doctor to a third party (e.g. a nurse or medical laboratory scientific officer), the third party must also sign that he or she has received the samples, giving the date and time (*see* Table 6.1 p. 107).

Forensic kits are usually supplied by the police force and the appropriate bags and labelling made clear. For samples sent to the laboratory for the identification of sexually transmitted infection, similar documentation is required.

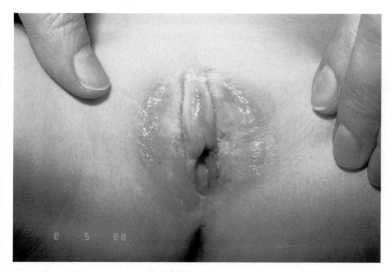

Figure 6.11 Lichen sclerosus complicated by streptococcal infection in a girl who was also abused

Table 6.6 Laboratory investigation for sexually transmitted organisms in the evaluation of sexually abused children

Gram staining of any genital or anal discharge

Cultures for *Neisseria gonorrhoeae* and *Chlamydia trachomatis*

Vaginal culture for *Trichomonas vaginalis* (girls)

Wet preparation for trichomonads and clue cells (girls)

Whiff test (girls)

Cultures of lesions for herpes simplex virus

Frozen serum sample

Serological tests for syphilis[a]

Hepatitis B surface antigen[a]

Human immunodeficiency antibody[a]

[a]If there is supportive epidemiological evidence.

KEY POINTS

1 Document carefully the history and examination findings. Be precise with terminology.
2 Avoid contaminating forensic evidence.
3 Inexperienced clinicians should refer possible child abuse cases to a doctor with specific expertise, such as a 'designated doctor for child abuse'.
4 Ensure that the correct samples are sent for an infection screen.
5 Draw up protocols locally for cases of possible sexual assault. Be sure to involve or include representatives from the relevant specialities: microbiology, paediatrics, A&E, gynaecology and genitourinary medicine.

chapter 7

SURGICAL ASPECTS OF VULVAL DISEASE

BASIC SURGICAL TECHNIQUES

PUNCH BIOPSY

Biopsy is indicated when the diagnosis is in doubt or if the management would be influenced by more information. An outpatient procedure with local anaesthesia is almost always both desirable and feasible. The choice lies between formal excision, convenient for some tumours, or a punch (Fig. 7.1) that may be used to

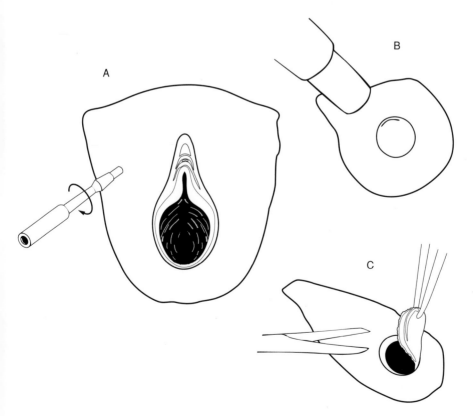

Figure 7.1 Punch biopsy of the vulva

remove completely very small lesions or to sample an area or a tumour. It is important to note on the request form to the pathologist exactly where the specimen has been taken from, since the histology varies from one part of the vulva to another. For example, the keratinized or non-keratinized epidermis, the presence or absence of skin appendages, and the clear glycogen-containing cells of the vestibule, which are easily mistaken for the koilocytes of a human papilloma virus infection need to be distinguished.

Procedure

The preliminary application of a eutectic mixture of prilocaine and lignocaine (Emla cream), left on for about 10 minutes with the thighs adducted, is helpful. No special skin preparation is needed, and clean but not necessarily sterile gloves will suffice. Lignocaine 1 per cent is then infiltrated, using a dental cartridge or a conventional syringe with a 30 gauge needle.

Disposable punches of 2–6 mm are chosen. The 6 mm size is used for larger lesions or when a biopsy is to be halved, one half being frozen for storage or sent for immunofluorescence. Some experience is required to become accustomed to the texture of the tissue compared with that of skin elsewhere, and to the angle of the surface; some advise practice on an orange or tomato.

The specimen is clearly defined by the punch in relation to the surrounding tissue and can, without trauma, be snipped off at the base with sharp scissors (Fig. 7.1c). Specimens for routine histology are then placed in a fixative, usually formol saline. Specimens for immunofluorescence should be rinsed in sterile saline and placed in a transport medium.

Haemostasis in the remaining defect can often be achieved with pressure and light cautery, but if preferred, and particularly when larger sized punches are used, an absorbable suture such as Vicryl 4000 is inserted. The patient is advised to wear a pad for the rest of the day. Further bleeding is rare, and healing is rapid.

Cervical biopsies will, when necessary, be taken by the gynaecologist or the physician in genitourinary medicine, again as an outpatient procedure. No local anaesthesia is required.

CRYOSURGERY

Tissue may be destroyed by extreme cold, at less than $-20°C$, because of the damage caused by intracellular ice crystals. A variety of agents can be used: liquid nitrogen $(-196°C)$, nitrous oxide $(-85°C)$ and carbon dioxide $(-70°C)$.

A small cryoprobe may offer successful treatment for mollusca contagiosa. The treatment of viral condylomas (genital warts) with several episodes of freezing and refreezing is often prolonged and painful. Cold can preserve the papilloma virus, and warts will often reappear if cryosurgery alone is used.

Cryosurgery should not be used on vulval or cervical intraepithelial neoplasia. It is, however, excellent for the treatment of cervical ectropion (an 'erosion').

LASER VAPORIZATION

Laser (Light Amplification by Stimulated Emission of Radiation) uses coherent light (parallel bundles of equal wavelength) beams of energy. Many surgical units use a laser beam produced by the excitation of carbon dioxide gas.

Tissue can be vaporized on impact, leaving the adjacent structures unaffected. The depth and size of destruction can be carefully controlled. This technique is ideally suited to the removal of multiple condylomas under general anaesthesia. Operators should wear mask protection as inhalation of the impact plume of smoke and steam may lead to nasal condylomas. Filtered suction extraction systems are essential.

Adequate biopsy is necessary to ensure accurate diagnosis before laser vaporization is used: lesions are reduced to a plume of vapour and are not available for subsequent histological scrutiny. It is this lack of availability of the excised lesion for pathological analysis that has led to the replacement of vulval and cervical intraepithelial laser vaporization treatment with electrodiathermy loop excision, or laser excision, which provides a complete specimen for histology and excellent healing.

Large and/or deep vulval lesions requiring extensive laser destruction may not heal as well as those treated by surgical excision and primary closure.

ELECTROSURGERY

High-frequency electrical wave energy causes the instant destruction of cells and can be used in two ways. Monopolar instruments do not require an 'indifferent' electrode plate in contact with the patient's thigh, whereas bipolar instruments do, the latter being used for both cutting and coagulation. They are extremely useful for stopping the intraoperative bleeding of small vessels and the fulguration (from the Latin for 'lightning') of condylomas.

The so-called Hyfrecator is often used in dermatological clinics. This is a high-frequency electrosurgical unit producing a low-voltage spark giving off only a small amount of heat. Often used in its monopolar mode, i.e. without the need for a ground plate attached to the patient, the electrode tip is placed on the lesion to produce electrodesiccation. If fulguration is required, the electrode is placed a few millimetres above the tissue to produce sparking between them. Small swellings such as condylomas can be removed, and basal cell carcinomas can be removed with a combination of desiccation and curettage. A short-angled needle is often used as the electrode tip, but loops, balls and wires are also available.

LOCAL EXCISION

The excision of vulval lesions by a small scalpel under local or general anaesthesia provides a specimen for pathological analysis (with clear edges) and an opportunity for good primary healing if an elliptical incision is used. If residual areas of atypia remain, these can be removed by further excision, which will still produce a good result.

The vulva has an excellent blood supply that, although occasionally troublesome during and after surgery, usually provides prompt and satisfactory healing. It is, however, necessary to produce good primary union of the skin edges without tension, and to close deeper spaces with multiple layers of sutures.

The skin edges may be approximated using fine dissolving sutures. Catgut has been used in the past, but many surgeons now use braided polyglycolic acid (e.g. Dexon), which is degraded by hydolysis. It loses the most of its breaking strength after 30 days, with complete absorption in 90–120 days. Braided polyglactin (e.g. Vicryl) is now frequently used in vulval surgery. It is twice as strong as catgut, and although it is more rapidly hydrolysed than polyglycolic acid (60–90 days), the inflammatory response it provokes is less. Some surgeons favour polydioxanone (e.g. PDS), which is a monofilament suture of great strength and is used where dehiscence may be likely.

STRUCTURAL DISORDERS: SPECIALIZED SURGICAL TECHNIQUES

IMPERFORATE HYMEN

Although a few babies are seen with hydrocolpos, most patients with an imperforate hymen are teenage girls presenting with primary amenorrhoea associated with cyclical pelvic pain. The retention of menstrual blood may produce a swelling (haematocolpos) large enough to cause urinary retention and/or a palpable abdominal mass. In cases of vaginal atresia, the mass may be felt per rectum and confirmed by ultrasound scanning. In most cases, clinical examination reveals a dark, bulging hymen.

The haematocolpos should not be lanced in the outpatient department – the quantity of altered blood obtained may be frightening to all concerned. Under general anaesthesia, a cruciate incision should be made under intravenous antibiotic cover. Redundant hymenal tissue should be excised to give a good functional and cosmetic result. Atresia of the lower third of the vagina may be managed by bringing down the upper two-thirds to the vulva after drainage of the haematocolpos.

RIGID HYMEN

A diagnosis of genuine hymen rigidus must be made after the exclusion of vaginismus as a cause of dyspareunia and/or difficulty in inserting a tampon. A rigid hymen may be semi-lunar or annular in appearance.

Treatment is by complete excision rather than random incision, being carried out under general anaesthesia. Great attention is paid to haemostasis; fine absorbable sutures are preferable to electrocautery, which may cause stenosis.

Vaginismus is a functional disorder, and patients with this condition are not usually helped by surgery, although they may occasionally require surgical examination under anaesthesia to exclude pathology.

HYMENORRHAPHY

Reconstitution of the hymenal remnants is occasionally requested for religious or social purposes prior to marriage. There are no medical indications for this procedure.

LABIAL FUSION

True fusion of the labia majora requiring surgical division under general anaesthesia is rare, although it may be seen in such conditions as ambiguous genitalia, for example in adrenogenital syndrome. Adhesions of the labia minora may occasionally occur in normal female infants but are easily separated with gentle care and rarely require surgery.

LABIAL REDUCTION

Enlargement of the labia minora, with or without fusion, may be seen in some forms of testicular feminization syndrome. Not infrequently, excessively large labia as a variant of normal are a cause of extreme embarrassment to teenage girls and those in early adult relationships.

Labial reduction can often bring pleasing results. However, the labia, like the rest of the vulva and mons, are extremely vascular, and meticulous care should be taken during surgery to ligature small vessels in order to prevent primary and secondary haemorrhage, infection and tissue breakdown.

CLITORAL HYPERTROPHY

An enlarged clitoris is found in those with ambiguous genitalia. When feasible, preventative hormonal manipulation is preferable to surgery. Clitoral amputation is not necessary, but reduction of the hypertrophied clitoris, with preservation of the glans and sexual sensation, requires considerable surgical skill and experience. Careful haemostasis may be difficult but is essential to achieve. Surgery may be required in reductive stages.

VULVOVAGINAL STENOSIS

Introital stenosis may occur in lichen sclerosus. Iatrogenic stenosis is relatively common. It follows the overzealous repair of an episiotomy after childbirth and may be associated with considerable pain and dyspareunia, especially if granulation tissue has occurred within the epithelial union or just beneath the scar. Stenosis may also occasionally occur after a colpo-perineorrhaphy operation for vaginal prolapse has been carried out incorrectly.

Procedures for the reconstitution of the perineum after episiotomy and plastic repairs should not be completed until an adequate introitus has been confirmed by digital examination. A proflavine-soaked vaginal pack left in place for 24 hours is helpful in large repairs in order to support the refashioned tissues and inhibit intravaginal adhesion formation. Further surgery may be avoided by the use of graded vaginal dilators, but badly healed episiotomy repairs often contain painful scar and granulation tissue, which needs to be excised before comfort can be restored.

Surgical treatment consists of excising all painful granulomatous inclusions and scar tissue. The introitus can be enlarged using a less radical form of Fenton's procedure (Fig. 7.2a–d), incising transversely along the fourchette, mobilizing the posterior vaginal wall for 2 or 3 cm above the incision, dividing the perineal scarring vertically down to, but not including, the muscles of the rectum (supported by a digit through the anal canal) and finally suturing the wound transversely.

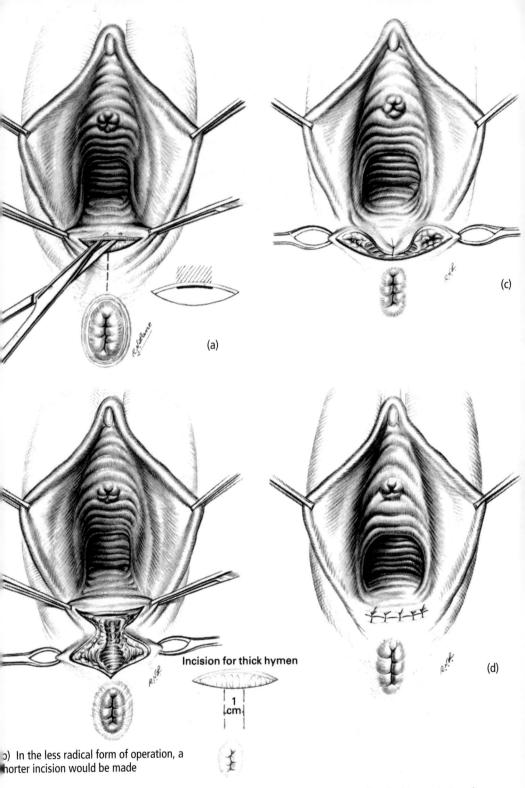

(a)

(c)

(b) In the less radical form of operation, a
shorter incision would be made

Incision for thick hymen

1 cm

(d)

Figure 7.2 Enlargement of the vaginal introitus: Fenton's procedure. (Reproduced with permission of
Arnold from Monaghan, J.M. (ed.) *Rob & Smith's Operative Surgery: Gynaecology and Obstetrics*, 4th
edn. Originally published in 1987 by Butterworth and Co. Ltd)

In many cases a vaginoplasty technique by way of a longitudinal incision 2 or 3 cm above the perineal skin and extending 2 cm below gives a better result, especially in failed episiotomy. The posterior vaginal epithelium and perineal skin is mobilized, paying great attention to haemostasis. Scarring can be excised and the superficial muscles of the perineum divided. The wound is then sutured transversely with interrupted sutures in order to widen the vulval opening to the desired degree. Vaginoplasty is especially helpful in lichen sclerosus, since the vaginal tissue does not subsequently become involved with the disease.

Such procedures should be carried out under general anaesthesia and intravenous antibiotic cover.

Vulvo-vaginal stenosis

In Stevens–Johnson syndrome, toxic epidermal necrolysis, erosive lichen planus and cicatricial pemphigoid adhesions often lead to partial or complete vaginal stenosis. The adhesions are removed by blunt dissection, care being taken to protect the rectum and urethra. Fusion may recur, and the risk of this must be minimized by the postoperative use of potent topical corticosteroids and vaginal dilators. Close co-operation between the gynaecologist and dermatologist is essential to provide optimal management.

VULVAL INJURY

The rich blood supply to the vulva often leads to large and very painful haematomas following closed injury, and to profuse haemorrhage after open laceration as well as, rarely, after first attempts at sexual intercourse. Haematomas may resolve with ice packs, patient elevation and an indwelling urinary catheter, in addition to general measures for shock, fluid replacement and possible antibiotic cover. In cases of open vulval injury, examination under anaesthesia may be necessary in order to facilitate the evacuation of a blood clot and the ligation of arterial bleeding. Bed rest and antibiotic prophylaxis will then be required. Resolution, while not being rapid, is usually complete and satisfactory.

NON-NEOPLASTIC SWELLINGS

Endometrioma

Excision is usually accompanied by laparoscopy to diagnose the extent of the endometriosis, and followed by 4–6 months of menstrual suppression therapy.

Urethral caruncle

A urethral caruncle is produced by a small prolapse of the distal urethral epithelium. It is often seen in the elderly, when it is frequently symptomless and may be left alone. Postmenopausal bleeding may be falsely attributed to it, so that the true cause, for example atrophic vaginitis or uterine carcinoma, is not discovered until later. If the caruncle is a source of bleeding, other causes have been excluded and the patient wishes to have it treated, it may be cauterized.

Bartholin's cyst

Surgery on an uninfected Bartholin's cyst is required when it becomes large enough to obstruct the introitus. Many cysts become infected, and the resulting abscess will need surgical intervention either when antibiotic therapy has failed or in cases of extreme pain and dyspareunia. Patients who have had abscesses that have burst and then reformed also benefit from marsupialization to produce better drainage. Marsupialization is always the preferred operation for Bartholin's abscess or cysts (Fig. 7.3). Excision of the gland is only required for extreme cases where multiple marsupialization procedures have failed. Excision may be associated with primary and secondary haemorrhage, residual pain and vaginal dryness, leading to frictional dyspareunia.

Marsupialization is carried out under general anaesthesia with the patient in the lithotomy position. The swollen gland is located and fixed with the thumb and forefinger (Fig. 7.3a). A vertical incision is then made to allow the new stoma to be placed where the blocked duct opened, i.e. on the vaginal side of the hymenal ring. Such an incision almost always heals in that site without scarring and subsequent dyspareunia.

Both the vaginal epithelium and the cyst wall are incised, and a small ellipse the size of the surgeon's finger diameter is removed. A sample of the cyst fluid and/or pus that emerges is sent for bacterial investigation on a dipstick swab. The forefinger is placed in the cyst cavity, and any loculations within the cyst are broken down digitally. All of the fluid is removed, and the edges of the cyst grasped with Littlewood's or Allis forceps.

A series of fine interrupted sutures is placed around the aperture, making sure that the vaginal epithelium is approximated to the cyst wall layers to ensure a draining gland without risk of stenosis and cyst recurrence (Fig. 7.3b). A drainage 'wick' should not be necessary if suturing is satisfactory.

NEOPLASMS

Vulval intraepithelial neoplasia

Vulval intraepithelial neoplasia (VIN) may also extend to the vagina (VAIN) and cervix (CIN) and/or down to the perianal margin (PAIN). In cases of PAIN, the anal canal should be thoroughly checked since extension may have occurred.

Originally treated by simple vulvectomy, i.e. excision of the labia and clitoris, VIN is now mainly managed by wide local excision. Local recurrence occurs in about 30% of patients treated by either method and may occur outside the field of a vulvectomy excision. Unlike the case with simple vulvectomy, the morbidity after local excision can be minimal, with preserved sexual function.

Laser vaporization of extensive areas of VIN may be followed by difficulty in healing, requiring skin grafting in exceptional cases. Postoperative pain is considerable compared with that seen in primary closure after surgical excision. Laser destruction must be of sufficient depth (between 3 and 5 mm) to destroy all

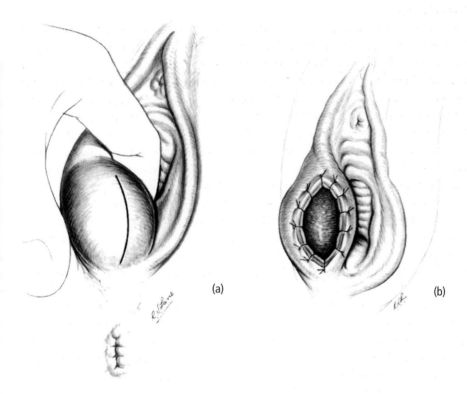

(a)

(b)

Figure 7.3 Marsupialization of a Bartholin's abcess or cyst. (Reproduced with permission of Arnold from Monaghan, J.M. (ed.) *Rob & Smith's Operative Surgery: Gynaecology and Obstetrics*, 4th edn. Originally published in 1987 by Butterworth and Co. Ltd)

of the VIN. Laser therapy may be inadequate in hairy areas where extension of disease down to the follicles may be missed. The lack of an excised specimen for histological scrutiny, which may reveal foci of invasive disease, makes laser vaporization unsatisfactory. The same shortcoming applies to topical 5-fluorouracil cream, this also being associated with little or no control over the depth and area of chemical destruction. Laser excision, using 'superpulse' lasers, has little if any advantage over surgical excision and primary suturing.

Extramammary Paget's disease

Wide local excision – to see whether there is an underlying adenocarcinoma – is advocated. When such a neoplasm is found, bilateral inguinal lymphadenectomy is necessary. In this condition, it is notoriously difficult to obtain disease-free margins. Micrographically controlled surgery may be of value. When surgery is not feasible, radiotherapy has a role. Small recurrences may be dealt with by non-surgical means (*see* Ch. 5).

Squamous cell carcinoma

An invasive carcinoma may present as a tumour or be discovered in areas of VIN that are quite flat. Many patients are elderly and may give a late presentation of advanced disease. Young and old patients with inguinal swellings should always have their genitalia carefully examined for a primary carcinoma.

The diagnosis must be confirmed by biopsy or excision before proceeding to definitive treatment. Whereas treatment protocols exist, much emphasis is now placed on the individualization of treatment, bearing in mind the size and site of the tumour, the degree of invasion, and the age and general health of the patient (see Ch. 5, Table 5.3).

When radical vulvectomy operations are indicated, they are performed using a wide variety of butterfly-type or separate incisions to permit groin node dissection and primary closure of the skin, with no tension, at the end of the operation, as, for example, in Fig. 7.4a–e. The vulvectomy may include part of the distal third of the urethra without loss of urinary continence, but care is required to avoid damage to the sphincter ani. Adequate suction drainage to remove large quantities of lymphoserous fluid, and prophylactic antibiotics, are required as wound breakdown is common. Early mobilization to prevent thromboembolism is important, as are effective support stockings to discourage lymphoedema. Such lymphoedema predisposes to recurrent attacks of cellulitis. Pre- and postoperative counselling may reduce psychological morbidity, especially in younger patients.

The few patients unsuitable for radical surgery may be offered irradiation.

Basal cell carcinoma

Surgical excision is the mainstay of treatment. Recurrences may occur, but micrographically controlled surgery may give superior results. This technique permits the controlled excision of tumours by the microscopic examination of horizontal sections cut from the periphery of an excision specimen, enabling the maximum preservation of normal tissue without leaving tumour behind. In practice, horizontal frozen sections are examined for residual tumour at the margins of excision so that further excision can be performed if necessary.

Malignant melanoma

If the diagnosis is not clear, the lesion should be excised with a narrow (2 mm) margin so that a full pathological assessment can be made. In the past, radical vulvectomy, incorporating excision with a wide (5cm) margin, and bilateral lymphadenectomy, was advocated for all malignant melanomas. Recent evidence suggests that, at the vulva as elsewhere, the prognosis depends mainly on the thickness of the tumour. This is preferably measured by the Breslow thickness, or alternatively by Clark's or Chung's levels, which correlate the depth of invasion with skin structures. There appears to be no advantage in achieving a margin of over 3 cm no matter how large the lesion. Bilateral lymphadenectomy is recommended where the melanoma is more than 0.75 mm in depth. New techniques to detect clinically occult metastases in the glands will be of value. Adjuvant therapy may also have a role. The possibility of distant metastases, for example in the liver and lungs, should be explored.

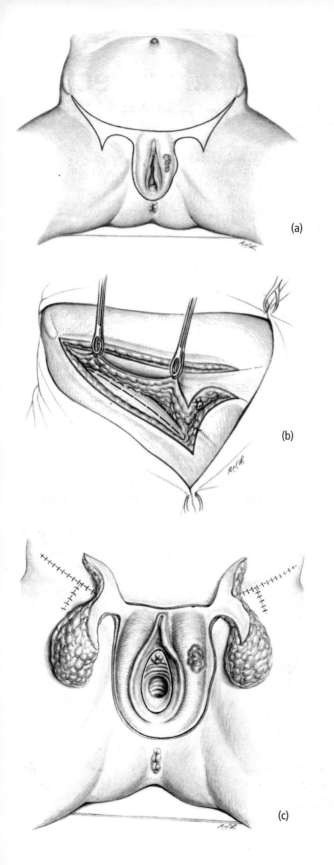

Figure 7.4 Radical vulvectomy. (Reproduced with permission of Arnold from Monaghan, J.M. (ed.) *Rob & Smith's Operative Surgery: Gynaecology and Obstetrics.* Originally published in 1987 by Butterworth and Co. Ltd)

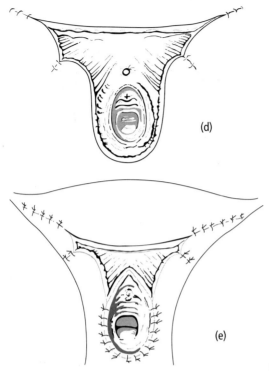

(d)

(e)

Figure 7.4 – *continued*

Carcinoma of Bartholin's gland

This is a rare tumour, occuring mainly in women between the ages of 40 and 55 years. It is often aggressive and highly malignant. A non-typical swelling in Bartholin's gland should be treated with suspicion. The tumour often presents as a hard, indurated swelling in the area of the gland, often associated with ulceration of the overlying skin.

Treatment, after confirmatory biopsy, is by radical vulvectomy and bilateral lymphadenectomy. However, the lymphatics from the Bartholin's glands drain into the anorectal glands, as well as into the inguinal glands, making complete excision difficult and the prognosis poor.

KEY POINTS

1 Any vulval lesion must be carefully examined and biopsy or excision will often be called for.
2 Carcinoma and precursors of carcinoma may masquerade as benign conditions.
3 Persistent or atypical-looking condylomas may be carcinomatous or precarcinomatous and should be biopsied.
4 Swellings in Bartholin's gland are not invariably benign.
5 Surgical treatment may be useful when epithelial disorders have led to stenosis.
6 The vulva has a rich blood supply; surgery may be complicated by primary or secondary haemorrhage if adequate care is not taken.

APPENDIX: SUGGESTIONS FOR FURTHER READING

Barton, S.E. and Hay, P.E. (eds) 1999. *Handbook of Genitourinary Medicine.* London: Arnold.

Champion, R.H., Burton, J.C., Burns, D.A. and Breathnach, S.M. (eds) 1998. Rook, Wilkinson & Ebling *Textbook of Dermatology.* 6th edn. Oxford: Blackwell Scientific Publications.

Department of Health, Education and Science. 1990. *Working Together. The Children Act 1989. A Guide to Arrangements for Inter-agency Cooperation for the Protection of Children from Abuse.* London: HMSO.

Eeedy, D.J., Breathnach, S.M. and Walker, N.P.J. 1996. *Surgical Dermatology.* Oxford: Blackwell Scientific Publications.

Fox, H. and Wells, M. (eds) 1995. *Haines and Taylor Obstetrical and Gynecological Pathology,* 4th edn. New York: Churchill Livingstone.

Holmes, K.K., Mardh, P-A., Sparling, P.F. and Wiesner, P.G. (eds) 1990. *Sexually Transmitted Diseases,* 2nd edn. New York: McGraw Hill.

Monaghan, J.M. (ed.) 1987. *Rob & Smith's Operative Surgery: Gynaecology and Obstetrics,* 4th edn. London: Arnold. Originally published by Butterworth and Co. Ltd.

Morse, S.A., Moreland, A.A. and Holmes, K.K. (eds) 1996. *Atlas of Sexually Transmitted Diseases and AIDS.* London: Mosby-Wolfe.

Ridley, C.M. and Neill, S.M. (eds) 1999. *The Vulva.* 2nd edn. Oxford: Blackwell Scientific Publications.

Royal College of Physicians of London 1997. *Physical Signs in Child Sexual Abuse,* 2nd edn. London: Royal College of Physicians.

Stokes, E.J., Ridgway, G.L. and Wren, M.W.D. 1993. *Clinical Microbiology.* 7th edn. London: Edward Arnold.

INDEX

Page numbers in **bold** refer to illustrations, those in *italics* refer to tables.